Severe Behavior Problems

Severe Behavior Problems
A Functional Communication Training Approach

V. MARK DURAND
State University of New York—Albany

Editor's Note by David H. Barlow

THE GUILFORD PRESS
New York   London

Printed in the United States of America

This book is printed on acid-free paper.

Last digit is print number: 9 8 7 6 5 4

Library of Congress Cataloging-in-Publication Data

Durand, V. Mark
    Severe behavior problems: A functional communication training
approach / by V. Mark Durand.
    p. cm. — (Treatment manuals for practitioners)
Includes bibliographical references and index.
ISBN 0-89862-206-9 (cloth)   ISBN 0-89862-217-4 (pbk.)
    1. Behavior disorders in children—Treatment. 2. Developmentally
disabled children—Rehabilitation. I. Title. II. Series.
RJ506.B44D85   1990
618.92'8914—dc20   90-44746
                                                                  CIP

Editor's Note

When behavior modification was young, which was not so many years ago, two dramatic developments attracted the field to this more "scientific" approach to behavior problems. The first was the apparent ability to treat phobia through systematic desensitization. The second was the potential of remediating severe behavior problems in children and adolescents, particularly severely disruptive and challenging behaviors. As with any new field, the success of these early approaches was overstated. Furthermore, aversive approaches to severe disruptive behavior stigmatized this new approach in the eyes of the public and public policy makers to the point where statutes to eliminate all behavior modification procedures were proposed in many legislatures.

Fortunately, behavior modification was not dependent on the charismatic appeal of the leader of a new "school" of psychotherapy, but rather on the tenets of science. With this in mind we began to carefully evaluate our results, pay attention to failures, and determine how we could do better.

Now, following years of intensive applied research, we have come to understand more deeply the nature and function of severely disruptive behavior. In this book Mark Durand presents, for the first time, a detailed manual on an alternative to aversive procedures for severely disruptive or challenging behavior. In tracing the development of these procedures Durand outlines the model of a scientific practitioner approach to problems with unfailing adherence to data-based evidence rather than intuition. In devising an effective data-based approach to the most severe of all behavior problems that does not rely on "aversives," Durand demonstrates convincingly the fulfillment of the lofty early goals of behavior modification and its founders to the benefit of all.

David H. Barlow
State University of New York—Albany

Preface

The purpose of this book is to describe a set of procedures used to reduce severe behavior problems—collectively referred to as functional communication training. It is *not* expected that someone will be able to pick up this book and, without prior training and experience, design and conduct a successful intervention plan for severe challenging behavior. Some background in the use of behavioral techniques with persons displaying severe disabilities is expected. However, it is hoped that this book will prove useful to practitioners of all types: teachers, paraprofessional staff, psychologists, speech and language therapists, and behavior analysts. Suggestions for assessment and intervention are provided for a broad range of problem behaviors. It is also hoped that sections of this book will be of interest to the parents, relatives, and friends of those who exhibit severe behavior problems. Instructors of advanced undergraduate and graduate students in psychology and special education may also find this book of value in courses covering behavior management.

The specific goals of the book include reinforcing the notion that an adequate conceptualization of any problem behavior is a necessary prerequisite to intervention. Without a model of behavior, intervention efforts will be nothing more than trial and error. One of many possible conceptualizations of challenging behavior is included here, and all subsequent assessment and intervention recommendations follow from this model. A second goal is to highlight the importance of an assessment prior to intervention. Specific assessment procedures are presented in an effort to improve the intervention design process. Certain assumptions are made in this book that influence the assessment approach provided. Other approaches may be equally valid, but do not necessarily follow the logic outlined here.

Organization

The remainder of this book is organized into four substantive sections: The first section is the Introduction, which outlines the use of terminology, certain assumptions held by the author, and the intervention philosophy that guides the assessment and treatment practices. The next section discusses a general model or conceptualization of problematic behavior. This model is offered to assist the process of assessment and treatment. It has always been an assumption that knowledge of the variables maintaining problem behavior is essential for successful intervention design, and the present conceptualization is offered to aid the information-gathering process. The third section describes the assessment of problem behavior. A review of the relevant literature is offered, along with a discussion of specific assessment procedures. Reinforcer selection is also discussed in some detail, because this is essential for the success of any intervention program, and because the activity has received increased attention in recent years.

The fourth section of the book describes the pertinent research and specific procedures involved in *functional communication training*. This intervention program has been the focus of much of our work over the years. However, with the exception of brief expositions in the Method sections of published research, these procedures and the rationales for many of the decisions made have never fully been described. Even when given the opportunity to present this work over 1- or 2-day workshops, the specific procedures and their rationales have only been introduced in a preliminary way. This book represents the first time all of this work has been collected in one place.

Functional communication training is an intervention package that includes both assessment procedures and intervention design. Therefore, it is essential that readers familiarize themselves with all aspects of the program. Skipping the assessment sections because "I know that material already" may lead to improperly matching intervention to the function of the problem behavior. On numerous occasions we have observed problems arising when teachers, parents, and clinicians assume they know what is maintaining a behavior, design an intervention based on this intuitive information, and the intervention subsequently failed. Was this a failure of the intervention? Maybe not. Such failures are occasionally due to improper assumptions about maintaining variables that are not based on systematic observation. It is strongly suggested, therefore, that even experienced readers consider the information in all of the sections in this book.

Quick Start

Workshop leaders and staff/teacher trainers may wish to direct participants in these training activities to only certain parts of this book. Trainees will get a good introduction to this approach by reading the case descriptions in Chapter 5 (Intervention Strategies). These case studies, when supplemented by an overview from a workshop leader, supervisor, or trainer, should provide a quick introduction to functional communication training. A more in-depth treatment of the material could include reading sections from Chapter 3 (Assessment) and Chapter 4 (Preintervention Considerations).

V. Mark Durand

Acknowledgments

Perhaps the most direct influence on the shaping of this book has come from two sources. The students who participated in the research projects and those for whom I have consulted have had a profound effect, and their efforts are greatly appreciated. Specifically, Elana, Greg, Jerry, Jewell, Jim, and Kathy have tested the limits of these procedures and to them I give a special thanks. In addition, I have had the privilege of conducting numerous workshops on these procedures over the past few years, and the participants in these workshops have challenged the procedures and their assumptions in a most constructive manner. Also, the Parsons Child and Family Center in Albany, N.Y., the Day Development and Transition Center of Brighton, Mass., the O.D. Heck Developmental Center in Schenectady, N.Y., the Mental Retardation Institute in Valhalla, N.Y., and the Suffolk Child Development Center of Smithtown, N.Y. have all opened their doors to our research efforts, and we are very grateful.

Grants from the Easter Seals Society and the National Institute on Disability and Rehabilitation Research have facilitated this work enormously. Specific efforts by Naomi Karp and Karen Faison have prodded me to disseminate this work to even wider audiences. Graduate students Jodi A. Mindell, Chris Kearney, Arleen Lanci, Jill Taylor, Marie Caulfield, and undergraduate students Debbie Todd, Susan London, Kathy Vays, Susan Schorr, David Salsburg, and Lisa Polidora have made valuable contributions to my thinking and work in this area and should be acknowledged. I owe an intellectual debt to my colleagues Luanna Meyer (who graciously reviewed an earlier draft of this manuscript), Dan Crimmins (who also co-authored the chapter on assessment), Paul Dores, Ted Carr, Ann O'Dea, Gloria Kishi, Frank Bird, Diana Moniz, and Jeff Robinson, without whom I would have made many more errors than are represented here.

USAir should be acknowledged for providing uninteresting settings in its airplanes and waiting areas that have on numerous occasions served as places to think and write. Most importantly, Wendy and Jonathan have supported these efforts above and beyond what should be expected from any family, and they have both my thanks and my love. Finally, I would like to dedicate this book to my parents (Julia and the late Vincent Edward Durand) for teaching me persistence and perhaps having more faith in me than I deserve.

Contents

1

Introduction

This book represents the culmination of more than a decade of clinical research with persons exhibiting severe behavior disorders. During this time, we endeavored to understand both these behavior problems as well as design assessment and intervention procedures to reduce or eliminate them. This process has rarely been easy, but has always been enlightening. Throughout these pages are the results of this educational experience—the successes and the failures of our efforts to help persons with severe behavior problems lead more independent and enjoyable lives.

The focus of the work—severe behavior problems—has taken a variety of forms. For example, there are times when these behaviors have been life-threatening. Some individuals have engaged in such severe forms of self-injurious behavior as to put their lives in danger. Additionally, other individuals have been so aggressive that parents and other caregivers have been fearful for their own safety. The severity of these challenging behaviors is also reflected in the intervention recommendations suggested by some. Excessively large doses of medication, prolonged isolation, surgery (e.g., removing teeth so that the person can't bite), and elaborate restraining/punishment procedures (e.g., tying a student to a table while in a helmet and spraying water in the face) are examples of the extremes to which such efforts have been taken.

More common, however, have been behaviors that are not life-threatening, but that significantly interfere with the quality of life of the persons engaged in these behaviors and for those with whom they live and work. Targets for these efforts include behaviors such as aggression (hitting, biting, scratching others), self-injurious behavior (head banging, hand biting, face slapping), tantrums (screaming, destroying objects), noninjurious stereotyped behaviors (hand flapping, rocking), and bizarre, psychotic speech.

Understanding and managing such problematic behavior continues to be a priority among persons who interact with individuals displaying severe disabilities. Behaviors such as aggression, self-injury, and tantrums are among the most frequently cited obstacles when attempting to place persons with handicaps in community settings (Eyman & Borthwick, 1980; Eyman & Call, 1977; Jacobson, 1982). Also, recidivism is increased significantly for those individuals leaving institutional settings if they exhibit such behaviors as aggression (Scheerenberger, 1981). Challenging behavior interferes with such essential activities as family life (Cole & Meyer, 1989), employment (Hanley–Maxwell, Rusch, Chadsey–Rusch, & Renzaglia, 1986; Hayes, 1987) and educational activities (Kerr & Nelson, 1989; Koegel & Covert, 1972). Additionally, such behaviors can pose a physical threat to these individuals and those who work with them. Problematic behavior compounds the already difficult task of improving the lives of persons with severe disabilities.

The consumers of our assessment and intervention efforts during this time have typically been described as having autism, mental retardation, and/or other severe developmental disorders. However, as will become clear, little additional information appears to be gained by emphasizing a correct diagnosis of these persons. Although it is important to know, for example, whether or not a person prefers the company of others, it does not appear useful when designing interventions to know whether or not a person has autism. A recent review of the literature reveals that the function of behavior problems and the outcomes of interventions for these behaviors may be similar for persons with a variety of diagnoses (Durand & Carr, 1989). Therefore, examples provided in the book will be drawn from experiences with persons exhibiting a number of different disorders.

Terminology

Throughout this book, words such as "consumers," "participants," "learners," or "students" are used to describe the individuals who have participated in our research program. These terms replace such words as "clients" or "subjects" because they are more descriptive of the roles they have played in the work. Additionally, terms such as "the mentally retarded" or "autistic children" are replaced with phrases such as "persons with mental retardation" and "children with autism" because this latter use emphasizes that they are people first, and only secondarily do they display various disabilities.

What follows is *not* (in the negative sense) a "cookbook." The assessment and intervention procedures being recommended are not meant to be exact and unvarying. As will become obvious, it is not unusual to make necessary modifications in these procedures to account for the differences in people and environments. Yet, in one sense, one could see the book as offering a variety of "recipes" (suggestions for assessment and intervention) that are designed to be experimented with and "seasoned to taste." It is hoped that readers will be exposed to a number of different approaches to assessment and intervention, which will, in turn, improve the delivery of services to the persons with whom we work.

Intervention Approach

Least Restrictive versus Rapid Suppression

There is an intervention approach that is adopted in this book that may be at variance with some recent positions espoused in the field. Perhaps the most widely accepted model is the "least restrictive alternative" model. This concept originated in the legal system, and suggests that interventions be introduced in order of their presumed restrictiveness, from least to most restrictive (Friedman, 1975; Guess, Helmstetter, Turnbull, & Knowlton, 1987; Shapiro, 1974; Turnbull, 1981; Zlotnick, 1981). More recently, a second model has appeared, which will be referred to as the "rapid suppression" model. In this approach, the speed with which an intervention may initially reduce the frequency of a problem behavior appears to be the criterion for use, even if it is an intervention that is highly intrusive. This view seems to usurp the least restrictive alternative model by eliminating the need to document the use of less restrictive procedures. A report by the Association for Behavior Analysis Task Force articulates this "rapid suppression" view quite explicitly.

> Consistent with the philosophy of least restrictive yet effective treatment, exposure of an individual to restrictive procedures is unacceptable unless it can be shown that such procedures are necessary to produce safe and clinically significant behavior change. It is equally unacceptable to expose an individual to a nonrestrictive intervention (or a series of such interventions) if assessment results or available research indicate that other procedures would be more effective. ... Thus, in some cases, a client's right to effective treatment may dictate the immediate use of quicker-acting, but temporarily more restrictive procedures. (Van Houten et al., 1988, pp. 113–114)

These recent statements seem to suggest that, independent of the seriousness of the behavior problem, more restrictive interventions are acceptable if one can *presume* that less restrictive alternatives would be ineffective. In 1982, the Association for the Advancement of Behavior Therapy Task Force took a similar, but more conservative approach to this philosophy when they addressed the treatment of self-injurious behavior.

On one hand, punishment, including very intense punishment such as shock, should
be considered for immediate inclusion in treatment: (a) in cases in which the client
is in imminent and extreme physical danger, or when the self-injurious behavior is
so intrusive as to prevent participation in habilitative and humanizing activities, or
(b) when "benign" procedures have been employed intensively and competently
and have not resulted in clinically significant improvement in self-injury. (Favell,
Azrin, et al., 1982, p. 542)

It is suggested that there are significant problems with this approach to
intervention, and that those working in this area should be cautious in
supporting this position. *A major problem with the rapid suppression philosophy is the implicit assumption that more restrictive equals more effective.*
Each of the positions outlined above implies that an argument can be made
for using more restrictive procedures in some cases because they might be
more effective. However, two recent, independent reviews of contemporary
empirical research suggest that degree of restrictiveness is *not* related to
effectiveness (Durand & Carr, 1989; Lennox, Miltenberger, Spengler, &
Erfanian, 1988). In many cases, less restrictive procedures were found to be
as good or better at reducing problem behavior when compared to more
restrictive interventions. In addition, a second assumption made in these
statements is that the severity of a problem behavior justifies the use of more
restrictive procedures. Again, however, there appears to be no logical or
empirical support for the assumption that restrictive procedures are more
effective than nonrestrictive interventions with severe challenging behavior
(Romanczyk, in press).

An additional problem with this approach stems from its conflict with
the accepted legal principles of "least restrictive alternative" or "least drastic
means." Individuals faced with defending the use of restrictive procedures
when less restrictive alternatives have not been tried or systematically
evaluated, may find their position at variance with legal precedents (e.g.,
Halderman vs. Pennhurst, 1977). Despite the apparent support from some
national organizations, those adopting this approach to intervention may find
their position difficult to defend, especially if they are required to argue this
approach in court.

A final problem with this position involves the ethical issues surrounding the use of intrusive and restrictive procedures on persons with severe
handicaps. Because many of these individuals can not give informed consent, the use of sometimes painful and stigmatizing interventions has been
denounced by professional organizations such as the Association for Retarded Citizens/US (ARC/US), the American Association on Mental Retardation
(AAMR), and the Association for Persons with Severe Handicaps (TASH,
1981), and individual professionals within the field (LaVigna & Donnellan,
1986; Meyer, & Evans, 1989; Sidman, 1989). A significant portion of those
working and living with persons exhibiting severe behavior problems argue

against the use of extremely restrictive interventions such as contingent electric shock *under any circumstances.*

Persons working in this field are confronted with a dilemma that may not go away. When faced with the charge of selecting an intervention procedure for a person exhibiting severe behavior problems, should they attempt less restrictive procedures in an expedient but comprehensive manner, or should they argue for going immediately to more restrictive procedures? The bias adopted here is for exhaustive efforts using less restrictive procedures, taking all possible precautions to protect everyone involved. This is a position that can be defended on empirical, legal, and ethical grounds.

Accommodation versus Assimilation

An additional aspect of the intervention philosophy adopted in this book involves what will be referred to as the "accommodation" versus the "assimilation" models of instruction (Durand, 1986a). An accommodation model involves changing the environment to fit the idiosyncratic needs of each individual. For example, if a person fails to learn how to tie shoes, one solution is to provide the person only with shoes that have velcro fasteners. Therefore, instead of spending years on this training, one may be able to change the environment to accommodate the student's difficulties. In an assimilation model of instruction, one attempts to help students adapt to current or future physical and social environments. For example, teaching students who are visually impaired to use a cane allows them to find their way independently, even in novel settings.

There appears to be a trend in special education toward an accommodation model for instructing persons with severe handicaps. It is important to note that an accommodation model of instruction is appropriate when possible *and* when the change does not create an overly artificial environment. However, concern is warranted when educators go to unusual lengths to set up trouble-free environments. These environments often differ substantially from the environment of "ultimate functioning" (Brown, Nietupski, & Hamre–Nietupski, 1976), and therefore could impose problems for transition. For example, we recently evaluated a program for a young man who would injure himself with combs. He would use the teeth of the comb to scratch up his arm, leaving open wounds. For the past few months, staff were reporting that this was no longer a serious problem. However, upon probing the situation, it became clear that the staff had become very good at making sure that all combs were constantly locked up. They reported that during those few times when they weren't vigilant, he would injure himself. Was his problem with self-injury solved?

Our approach is primarily one of assimilation. Using the example from above, a different approach would have been to assess *why* the young man was injuring himself with combs, and to attempt to address his behavior problem with skills training. An assessment of his self-injury might indicate, for example, that he scratched himself to escape from difficult tasks. Using functional communication training, we would teach him to request assistance or a break from work. Therefore, instead of artificially removing the opportunity to engage in the behavior (accommodation), or removing all tasks that may be difficult (accommodation), he would be taught an appropriate reaction to difficult tasks (assimilation). Throughout the book examples will be given of the judicious use of both accommodation and assimilation strategies that attempt to facilitate the placement of students in less restrictive settings.

Assumptions

In order to aid the intervention process, we have spent a great deal of time looking for reasons that individuals continue to engage in these problem behaviors. Guiding our efforts to understand these behaviors better has been an implicit assumption; that *such behavior problems are not abnormalities. Instead, these responses are reasonable behavioral adaptations necessitated by the abilities of our students and the limitations of their environments.* Therefore, we have looked to the environment and its effect on the behaviors of our consumers.

Implied by this approach is a downplaying of the role of physiological variables in the *maintenance* of these behaviors. It is recognized that physiological influences must play a part, especially in the origins of these behaviors (Cataldo & Harris, 1982). Unfortunately, however, to date there has been relatively little systematic research on the specific influence that genetics and biology play on problem behavior. In contrast, there have been numerous studies documenting the role of social and physical variables on these behaviors. We have assumed that most of these behaviors *continue to be exhibited* because of the effects they create on the behaviors of others and in their physical surroundings (for some exceptions, see Chapter 2). We continue to test this assumption through our work.

Scientist–Practitioner Model

As has been mentioned above, this book describes assessment and intervention procedures that are developed from a program of research lasting more than a decade. The goal has always been to emulate a "scientist-practitioner" model, with our work being data-based and ultimately directed by our data (Barlow, Hayes, & Nelson, 1984). However, also discussed are clinical-educational issues that, at times, go beyond the data we and others have generated. There have been literally thousands of clinical decisions made over the years that have not been systematically investigated. We have tried at all times to be empirical in our approach—evaluating the outcomes of these decisions. But it is recognized that work is not finished in this area. Whenever possible, an attempt is made to distinguish between tested and validated procedures from those that have seemed to work with one or two students. For example, the discussion of interventions for sensory-maintained behavior problems is based on a few clinical trials, and not on extensive, controlled research. Such recommendations are included because (1) It is believed they can be helpful to educators and clinicians, and (2) It is hoped that others will assist in investigating this package of procedures.

Throughout this book, those occasions where our efforts have failed are described. Although obviously difficult for anyone working as a researcher/clinician/educator, we have tried to remain critical of our own work and its outcomes. It is often the case that attention to the failures and the processes underlying them has brought about a greater understanding of the persons with whom we work and their behavior. Some of our better work seems to follow major breakdowns in our most carefully designed plans.

Beyond Communication Training

This book provides a detailed, descriptive account of how to implement one, albeit important, aspect of intervention. Teaching alternative communication strategies should be an important part of any plan to reduce problem behavior. It will become clear that there is no attempt here to provide a comprehensive account of all possible interventions. Rather, we have attempted to discuss one approach thoroughly. It should be recognized, however, that a total intervention plan for any presenting problem should involve a comprehensive strategy for changing numerous aspects of the person involved, relevant other persons, and the surrounding environment (Meyer & Evans, 1989). Whenever possible and appropriate, this book addresses these issues in the context of the communication training. For example, is the environment in which the person is attempting to communicate adequate? Is the person provided with options or choices, especially when they are requested? *More often than not, the environment experienced by persons with severe disabilities—especially those with challenging behavior—reflects a substandard life-style that we ourselves would find unacceptable.* Readers will be directed to the writings of others that more thoroughly address issues such as altering programs, environments, and even life-styles when these changes are clearly needed.

Compatibility with Applied Behavior Analysis

Readers will note that, at times, some of the recommendations made here will appear to conflict with accepted behavioral practices (e.g., how to respond to problem behavior). These departures, however, typically stem from how some educators and clinicians have *interpreted* behavioral principles and translated them into intervention strategies. For example, workers in this area typically assume that praise is a universal reinforcer, and routinely incorporate praise as a consequence for all appropriate responses. However, as will be seen in the section on reinforcer assessment, praise can serve as a neutral or even an aversive consequence for some individuals. The suggestions for selecting and using reinforcers, as well as other interventions, are consistent with traditional behavioral principles, although they may at times conflict with current common practice.

These are exciting times for workers in the area of developmental disabilities. Important issues such as community integration (Meyer & Putnam, 1988), teaching children with handicaps in regular versus special educational settings (Brown et al., 1989a, 1989b), and the use of procedures employing aversive stimuli (Guess et al., 1987) have at times polarized the field. However, these controversies have also motivated some stimulating discussion and research that will ultimately lead to the improvement of services for persons with severe handicaps. It is hoped that this book will in some way contribute to this process and further the efforts of the legions of persons who daily assist people with handicaps to lead more productive and fulfilling lives.

2

Severe Behavior Problems

"It's not what you say, but how you say it."

Before discussing specific assessment and intervention strategies, it is important to outline influences that significantly impact on challenging behavior. A review of the research on these influences or controlling variables is presented in this chapter, as well as a proposed model of problem behavior. This model has provided the foundation for functional communication training and has been heuristic in the development of the procedures used in this work. A review of the intervention literature particularly relevant to this work will then be presented, accompanied by a discussion of this approach to behavior problems and how it affects intervention design.

Influences on Problem Behavior

Undoubtedly, there are an unlimited number of stimuli that can and do influence problem behavior. A plethora of events has been assessed to influence problem behavior, including such things as group density (e.g., Hutt & Vaizey, 1966; Repp, Barton, Gottlieb, 1983), relocation (e.g., Cohen, Conroy, Frazer, Snelbecker, & Spreat, 1977), lighting conditions (e.g., Colman, Frankel, Ritvo, & Freeman, 1976), adaptive clothing (e.g., Rojahn, Mulick, McCoy, & Schroeder, 1978), social attention (e.g., Lovaas, Freitag, Gold, & Kassorla, 1965), tangible consequences (e.g., Durand & Crimmins, 1988), escape from unpleasant events (e.g., Carr, Newsom & Binkoff, 1976), and sensory consequences (e.g., Rincover & Devany, 1982). This abridged list highlights only a few of the vast array of influences that have been observed to affect the problem behavior of some individuals.

Despite this impressive listing, an additional assumption implicit in our work is that there are a limited and circumscribed number of *important* classes of maintaining variables. Although it is probably true that for any one individual a great number of stimuli control his or her behavior, it is presumed that meaningful influence is exerted by only a small number of these stimuli. This assumption has both practical and empirical origins. If it were true that one needed to assess a virtually unlimited number of stimuli that control the behavior of students, then such an assessment process would clearly be impractical. A complete analysis of this type could last for months, and occupy the time and effort of a large number of concerned persons. Fortunately, recent research suggests that there are a limited number of powerful stimuli or classes of stimuli that appear to influence the behavior of a large number of students exhibiting problem behavior (Carr, 1977; Durand & Carr, 1985). And, the present focus on those influences that significantly affect behavior problems is consistent with the concern of applied behavior analysis with the practical importance of such analyses (Baer, Wolf, & Risley, 1968).

What follows is a brief review of the research on maintaining variables, and an outline of one model of problem behavior. It will become apparent that the proposed model does not include all of the possible variables controlling problem behavior. Given our assumption about these behaviors, we have purposely limited the model to those influences that appear to exert strong control over the problem behavior of a large number of students.

Stimulus Events

Stimulus events are those influences that are simple, discrete, and immediate. One example of a stimulus event might be a parent saying "Put your hands down!" when a young boy bites his hand. This is in contrast with "setting events," which are more complex conditions that may be concurrent with the behavior problem or more distant in time (Bijou & Baer, 1961; Wahler & Fox, 1981; a separate review of setting events is included below). Although there has been disagreement over the precise use of these terms (see, for example, Goldiamond, 1983; Leigland, 1984; Michael, 1982), they will be adopted here as defined above for purposes of discussion.

There are a number of categorization systems that have been proposed for stimuli possibly affecting behavior problems. Some models limit the classes of important stimuli to two or three (e.g., Carr, 1977), although others have expanded this to more than 30 (e.g., Donnellan, Mirenda, Mesaros, & Fassbender, 1984). Empirical evidence for a large number of important influences on behavior problems is lacking, although parallels with the functions of nonverbal communication suggest alternative ways of looking

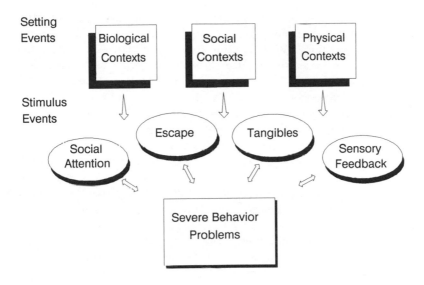

FIGURE 2-1. A model of the classes of stimuli influencing severe behavior problems.

at these influences that may lead to finer distinctions (see discussion below in the section on "Problem Behavior as Communication").

We have adopted an empirical/heuristic approach to classifying controlling variables. In other words, classes of stimuli have been culled from the research literature with an eye toward groups of stimuli that could be usefully translated into interventions. As seen in Figure 2-1 and in the review below, four classes of stimulus events have been identified for purposes of assessment and teaching alternative communicative responses. Again, there are other ways of grouping these influences, but our experience has shown this organization to be particularly helpful in designing interventions for severe behavior problems.

SOCIAL ATTENTION

Some of the earliest work in this area suggested that problem behavior in some individuals may be shaped and maintained by social attention as a consequence. In other words, some challenging behavior may be positively reinforced by the attention of others. In a now classic study by Lovaas and colleagues (Lovaas et al., 1965), empathic statements (e.g., "I don't think you are bad!") were presented to a 9-year-old girl each time she hit herself.

This presumably humanistic treatment resulted in an *increase* in her self-injurious behavior, indicating that attention from others may have been reinforcing her behavior. Withdrawing social attention (i.e., extinction), contingent upon her self-injury, decreased the frequency of this behavior.

Martin and Foxx (1973) employed a form of social isolation in an effort to assess and intervene on the aggressive behavior of one woman with retardation. An experimenter sat in the room alone with the woman. During one phase of the study, the experimenter ignored the woman's aggressive behaviors. The noncontingent social isolation resulted in significant decreases in aggression. A second phase was then introduced in which the experimenter responded verbally following each instance of aggression (e.g., "How can you behave that way?"). This contingent attention prompted an increase in aggressive episodes. Returning to ignoring again resulted in decreased aggression. These and subsequent investigations have pointed to social attention as a variable maintaining some problem behavior (e.g., Carr & Durand, 1985b; Carr & McDowell, 1980; Durand, 1984; Lovaas & Simmons, 1969). In other words, behaviors such as self-injury and aggression may continue to be exhibited because they are positively reinforced by the attention of others.

This is important work, because it suggests that behaviors such as bizarre self-injury (e.g., head banging, hand biting) and aggression can serve a useful function for an individual (i.e., eliciting social attention). It is also important from an intervention standpoint. For many, it is very natural to come to the aid of someone who is upset. For example, if we see a child crying or in pain, it is likely that we would want to pick up the child, hold him or her, and otherwise provide comfort. However, the previous research points out that for some individuals such "loving care" can actually be harmful. Social attention can have negative effects if it becomes a regular consequence for these troubling behaviors, and especially if hugs and attention are almost *never* given to the child otherwise.

TANGIBLE CONSEQUENCES

In addition to social attention, tangible consequences (e.g., food, toys, activities) may also serve as positive reinforcement for these behaviors. Evidence for the role of tangibles comes from research showing that problem behavior can increase following contingent access to preferred play activities (Lovaas & Simmons, 1969) and following the initial withdrawal of tangible reinforcers (Durand, 1986b; Durand & Crimmins, 1988; Edelson, Taubman, & Lovaas, 1983; Horner & Budd, 1985). Problem behavior may be maintained in some individuals by the tangible consequences resulting from these behaviors (Doss, 1988; Doss & Reichle, 1989; Durand & Carr, 1985; Durand & Crimmins, 1988).

Again, important implications for intervention are evident. For example, suppose a student regularly was aggressive in order to obtain certain tangible consequences (e.g., going outside and playing on the swings). In this case, if a teacher or parent chose not to attend to a behavior problem (e.g., they turned and walked away) but still allowed a student to gain access to a favorite tangible as a consequence for problem behavior (e.g., could go outside and play to "calm down"), then it would tend to reinforce the problem behavior. Even though the caregivers thought they were removing a reinforcer (attention), they may have inadvertently delivered a potent reinforcer contingent on problem behavior (i.e., access to the swings).

ESCAPE

Negative reinforcement has also been explored as a process involved in the continued presence of problem behavior. In other words, some individuals may engage in these behaviors to remove themselves from aversive situations. Several studies have demonstrated that behavior problems will increase following the introduction of presumably aversive stimuli (e.g., difficult task items) (Carr & Durand, 1985a; Carr, Newsom, & Binkoff, 1976, 1980; Churchill, 1971; Durand, 1982b; Romanczyk, Colletti, & Plotkin, 1980; Weeks & Gaylord–Ross, 1981).

In this case, some students may learn that if they want demands or other unpleasant situations to end, then engaging in problem behavior will serve this purpose. For example, suppose a father asks his daughter to make her bed. However, instead of making her bed, she yells, screams, and falls to the floor. After a number of requests (and some yelling), the father decides to leave saying "I'll come back when you calm down." Later, the father comes back and makes the bed himself. In this case, the daughter may have learned that by engaging in tantrums she could get her father to stop making demands on her. She was negatively reinforced for misbehaving by the father's withdrawal of aversive demands (see Patterson, 1982, for a thorough discussion of this type of interaction pattern).

SENSORY FEEDBACK

In addition to the socially mediated variables just described, the sensory consequences provided by some problem behaviors (e.g., auditory, visual, tactile) have been suggested as possibly involved in their maintenance.

Challenging behavior for some individuals may continue because the sensory feedback it provides is reinforcing. Reductions in problematic behavior assumed to be maintained by its sensory consequences has been accomplished through removing these consequences (Rincover & Devany, 1982), masking them (Durand, 1982b), or by providing alternative ways of obtaining this sensory feedback (Favell et al., 1982).

One of the major implications for intervening with behaviors maintained by their sensory consequences has to do with withholding social attention. Ignoring such behaviors should have no effect, because they are essentially "self-reinforcing." Even though ignoring is one of the first interventions attempted with behavior problems, this type of reaction can probably be ruled out immediately with behaviors being maintained by their sensory consequences.

MULTIPLE INFLUENCES

The previous discussion indicates that the problematic behavior of different individuals may be maintained by different consequences. Although one individual's self-injury may be maintained by its positive social consequences (e.g., additional adult attention), another individual's self-injury may continue to occur because it results in the removal of demands (e.g., academic tasks), provides access to tangibles (e.g., toys), or furnishes sensory input (e.g., auditory feedback). However, problem behavior *within* individuals may also be maintained by different consequences. For example, in one study we found that although two topographies of self-injury (head hitting and face hitting) exhibited by a boy with severe handicaps were maintained by their sensory consequences, one of these behaviors, face hitting, was also influenced by increased task difficulty (Durand, 1982b). One interpretation of this study is that at times the boy hit himself because it felt good. However, it may also have been the case that he learned that if he hit himself in the face, those who worked with him would "back off" on any demands. This reaction by others to his face slapping could have served to negatively reinforce face hitting in some situations (e.g., when he was asked to do something he didn't want to do). Intervention, therefore, would need to address both the sensory nature of his face hitting, along with the possibility that he would sometimes use the behavior to escape unpleasant situations.

Although there are relatively few systematic investigations of the nature of behavior problems for particular students in a variety of settings, it would be safe to assume that over time some students learn to use their behavior problems for a variety of purposes (e.g., to gain attention, to gain access to tangibles) (Durand & Carr, 1987). It appears that problem behavior *between* and *within* individuals may be multiply determined (Carr, 1977; Durand, 1982; Durand & Carr, 1985; Iwata, Dorsey, Slifer, Bauman, & Richman, 1982).

Setting Events

Recall that *setting events are complex conditions that occur concurrent with problem behaviors or are more distant in time* (Bijou & Baer, 1961; Wahler & Fox, 1981). For example, one setting event might include getting a bad night's sleep the day before an episode of aggression. To date, there has been little systematic research exploring the complete range of possible setting events that is comparable to the work with stimulus events. Yet, there have been numerous studies that have correlated changes in behavior problems as a function of concurrent or temporally distant global changes in the internal or external environment. Because many of these influences will impact on intervention decisions, this work will be briefly reviewed below.

PHYSIOLOGICAL CONTEXTS

One of the most common explanations for the continued occurrence of problem behavior in students involves physiological hypotheses. Behavior problems have been attributed to a variety of illnesses and other abnormal biological conditions (Cataldo & Harris, 1982). Despite the prevalence of such explanations, relatively little research has focused on the influence of physiological variables on problem behavior. This is probably due to the obvious difficulty in studying this phenomenon. For example, such influences can rarely be manipulated (e.g., making a student ill); thus experimental analyses tend to be problematic. Also, because it is difficult to predict just when certain physical conditions will occur, even correlational research can be difficult.

Fortunately, however, some data are available on a few physiological influences. Gedye (1989) recently hypothesized that extreme self-injury among some individuals may be attributed to frontal lobe seizures. Only indirect support for this theory was provided, and a direct test of this hypothesis awaits verification. Another physiological condition, the hormonal changes associated with puberty, has been hypothesized to influence problem behavior. Gillberg and Steffenburg (1987), for example, observed that challenging behavior in children with autism was reported to become more serious following puberty.

Pharmacological interactions can also play a part in the presence of challenging behavior. For example, we observed that for one young man, severe self-injurious behavior was less frequent when both a behavioral intervention and medication were employed (Durand, 1982a). When either the behavioral intervention or the medication (haloperidol) was removed, his self-injury increased. It was hypothesized that the medication served to make the behavioral intervention more effective. Podboy and Mallery (1977) observed that by decreasing caffeine in the coffee consumed by the residents of one program, there was a corresponding decrease in aggressive outbursts.

Organic influences have been examined with respect to their role in the etiology and maintenance of problem behavior such as self-injury (Carr, 1977; Cataldo & Harris, 1982). Such conditions as Lesch–Nyhan syndrome, Cornelia de Lange syndrome, and otitis media have been associated with problematic behavior in some individuals. This association does not negate, however, the role of the social and sensory consequences just discussed. For example, self-injury in persons with Lesch–Nyhan syndrome has been shown to be amenable to change following behavioral treatments (e.g., Duker, 1975). In addition, self-injury of organic origin may acquire social functions by way of interactions with parents, teachers, and other caregivers (Carr & McDowell, 1980). Again, most of the research in this area has been, by necessity, correlational. Therefore, the exact influence of many of these physiological variables is difficult to assess.

SOCIAL CONTEXTS

The data on social contexts also lack a cohesive model. The research in this area has mostly involved single demonstrations that have not been systematically replicated. The contexts that have been studied vary from widespread administrative contexts, to more molecular influences. For example, our work in the area of employee absenteeism policies demonstrated a possible link with challenging behavior (Durand, 1983, 1985). We observed that as absenteeism decreased following a change in policy, the students were also observed to decrease their problem behavior. When absenteeism increased following a reversal of the policy, problem behavior also increased (Durand, 1983).

Gardner, Cole, Davidson, and Karan (1986) found that the aggressive behavior of one young man was affected by a variety of setting events. For example, they observed that aggressive outbursts were more likely to occur following home visits with his brother present and the presence of a male staff member. They concluded that these types of setting events interacted with his responses to the stimulus events occurring during the day (e.g., corrective feedback, staff prompts). In other words, he was more likely to become aggressive following corrective feedback on those days following a home visit where his brother was present.

A number of investigators have explored behavioral contrast as a setting event affecting problem behavior. Behavioral contrast is a "change in the rate of responding during the presentation of one stimulus in a direction away from the rate of responding prevailing during the presentation of a different stimulus" (Reynolds, 1961). For example, Lovaas and Simmons (1969) used contingent electric shock to reduce the frequency of self-injurious behavior in three children with mental retardation. Successful reductions in self-injury for two of the children in the presence of one experimenter produced concomitant increases in self-injury in the presence of other adults. Although there have been occasional observations of behavioral contrast (e.g., Koegel, Egel, & Williams, 1980; Wahler, 1975), this area warrants more systematic study.

In related research, we observed that students with problem behavior maintained by escape from task demands responded differently to demands, depending on the task presented previously (Durand & Carr, 1982). In other words, if a moderately difficult task was preceded by an easy task, then the student was likely to engage in more problem behavior during the moderately difficult task (presumably to escape the task). On the other hand, if the task was preceded by a more difficult task, then the student was less likely to display problem behavior. This study showed that the conditions just preceding the events correlated with problem behavior can affect its occurrence.

PHYSICAL CONTEXTS

A variety of physical contexts have been correlated with the occurrence of challenging behavior. It should be noted that physical contexts and the often-associated change in social contexts are frequently not separated when they are studied. For example, problem behavior has been observed to increase with physical crowding, although there are a variety of social interactional changes that can take place in such settings as well (Hutt & Vaizey, 1966; Repp et al., 1983) Conclusions, therefore, about the relative effects of physical versus social contexts should be viewed cautiously.

Wearing certain clothing has been observed to decrease self-injurious behavior in some individuals (Rojahn et al., 1978). Noise levels have often been hypothesized to affect problem behavior, yet outside of infant research (e.g., Brackbill, Adams, Crowell, & Gray, 1966), very little research is available on this setting event. Various physical arrangements have also been suggested as possibly influencing these behaviors, but again, little experimental evidence is available (Forness, Guthrie, & MacMillan, 1982). Physical relocation has been studied in the context of deinstitutionalization, and a variety of studies have shown generally positive effects with individuals displaying severe disabilities (e.g., Cohen, Conroy, Frazer, Snel-becker, & Spreat, 1977; Conroy, Efthimiou, & Lemanowicz, 1982; Schroeder & Henes, 1978; Singer, Close, Irvin, Gersten, & Sailor, 1984).

DIRECTION OF EFFECTS

As Figure 2-1 illustrates, our model (and those of others, e.g., Gardner et al., 1984) assumes that setting events do not have a direct effect on problem behavior. Instead, such conditions as illness, sleep disorders, group density, staffing patterns, and temperature effect the salience of the stimulus events. In other words, being tired will not make you severely self-injurious. How-ever, being tired when someone places heavy demands upon you will more likely make you react to those demands. Similarly, having an earache will not make you aggressive. Yet, if someone you like is ignoring you when you are in pain, you would be more likely to respond.

This interpretation suggests that although setting events are extremely important, you also need to know the specific stimulus events under which behavior problems are more likely to occur. This has direct implications for treatment. For example, although you may not be able to eliminate an earache immediately, you could teach the student to request a break from work in order to rest. Our recommendation is always to assess and screen for possible setting events. However, when these are not readily apparent, or they are not amenable to change (e.g., puberty) it does not mean that you cannot inter-vene. We will illustrate the specific intervention steps in Chapter 5.

Reciprocal Influences

As the arrows in Figure 2-1 suggest, we are hypothesizing that stimulus events influence problem behavior, *and* problem behavior can influence stimulus events. In other words, *there is a reciprocal relationship between problem behavior and the environment.* How people behave toward you can, for example, contribute to your aggression, and your aggression can change how people behave toward you. Although rarely discussed in writings about persons with severe handicaps, workers in the area of child development have long recognized that children are not only influenced by their environ-ment but also have an effect on it (Bell, 1968; Rheingold, 1969; Shatz & Gelman, 1973; Snow, 1972).

Despite the large number of studies focusing on the behavior problems of persons with severe handicaps, until recently none has systematically explored the reciprocal relationship between these behaviors and the be-

havior of parents, teachers, or others. Our research has explored how behaviors such as self-injury influences teachers. In one preliminary study, we
found that the severe self-injury of one adolescent girl (Kate) was influenced
by social attention, and the self-injury of one young man (Jim) was influenced by escape (Durand, 1986b). Figure 2-2 shows the data on *teacher
behavior* toward these two students. Although there was little difference in
the percentage of comments (i.e., neutral expressions) or praise toward these
two students, there was a difference in the percentage of time spent with each
of them (proximity) and the percentage of commands (requests to perform
activities). It appeared that teachers spent more time with and asked more of
Kate then they did with Jim.

These data suggest that Kate's attention-getting self-injury may have
been successful in soliciting teacher attention in the form of proximity and
commands. From the teachers' perspective, Kate may be better behaved if
they are close to her and give her more work to accomplish. On the other
hand, Jim's behavior appeared successful in removing himself from most
interactions. Teachers might inadvertently be reinforced with reductions in
his self-injury by leaving him alone most of the day.

These and other data (see Durand & Kishi, 1987) are beginning to point
out that those who interact with persons exhibiting severe behavior problem
are also influenced by these responses. And, this influence can at times have
a negative impact on such activities as teaching. For example, although Kate
and Jim were relatively well behaved during most of their instructional day,
as seen above, Kate required almost constant attention, and Jim was not
engaging in any educational programming. These results suggest that such
reciprocal relationships should be assessed, and potential problem interactions may need to be addressed.

The overall model just presented suggests that behavior problems serve
a function for those who engage in them. This has led to hypotheses about
the possible relationship between challenging behavior and communication.
In what follows, we will review the evidence for such a relationship, and
discuss the value of such a hypothesis.

Problem Behavior as Communication?

The idea that problem behavior may serve as a form of communication has
a long history (Carr & Durand, 1985b). Crying by children, in particular, has
frequently been viewed as an attempt to communicate. Anyone who has
observed a crying child and a frantic parent trying to discover what the child
seems to want is struck by the power of this behavior. The earliest recorded
observations support this notion. Plato observed that the crying seen in

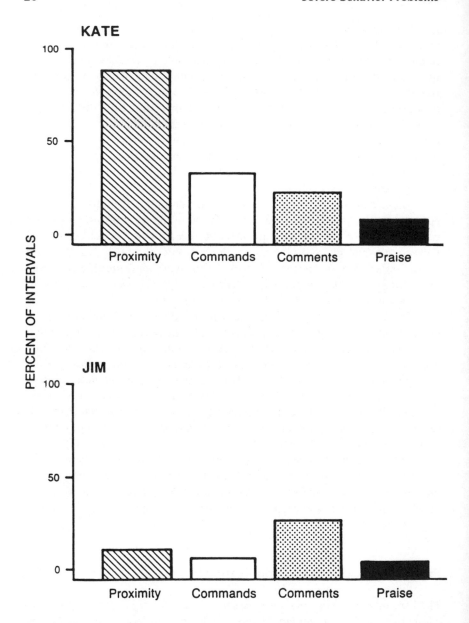

FIGURE 2-2. Mean rates of adult attention and proximity by staff toward Kate and Jim. From "Self-injurious Behavior as Intentional Communication" (p. 152) by V. M. Durand, in K. D. Gadow, Ed., *Advances in Learning and Behavioral Disabilities* (Vol. 5), 1986, Greenwich, CT: JAI. Copyright 1986 by JAI Press, Inc. Reprinted by permission of the authors and publisher.

infants may be an attempt to get caregivers to fulfill their desires (Plato, 348 B.C./1960, p. 174). Rousseau also observed that crying may have communicative properties (1762/1979, p. 77). Family systems theorists have long relied on the idea that nonverbal behavior has communicative properties (e.g., Haley, 1963; Minuchin, 1974). And, over the last two decades, developmental psychologists have systematically studied the communicative nature of nonverbal behavior in young children (Bates, Camaioni, & Volterra, 1975; Bruner, 1973; Wolff, 1969).

The hypothesis that behavior has functions served as the basis for early theorizing about behavior. For example, the functionalists, such as William James (1893), suggested that mental processes evolved to serve useful functions for individuals struggling to cope with complex environments (Rachlin, 1970). Early behaviorists also emphasized the functional nature of problem behavior. These workers did not see problem behavior as only excesses requiring suppression. They hypothesized that these actions were rational and reasonable reactions to antecedents and consequences present in the internal and/or external environment. Ferster (1965), for example, described the situations surrounding a child's crying:

"Crying could occur as a reflex effect of a loud noise, a temperature extreme, or food deprivation. Or it could result from a parental reaction providing consequences to the child, which, in turn, increases the frequency of crying" (p. 10).

The previous review of stimulus and setting events illustrated that problem behavior exhibited by persons with severe developmental disabilities can, like communication, serve multiple social functions. And, the idea that the problem behavior of persons with severe handicaps can serve a communicative function has intuitive appeal. These persons characteristically have difficulty communicating their wants and needs. Parents and other caregivers often describe persons with severe and multiple handicaps as being "frustrated" because they appear to want to communicate but can't. Correlational research in this area also appears to support this idea. For example, Talkington, Hall, and Altman (1971) observed that aggression was more prevalent among persons with severe communication difficulties. Similarly, persons most likely to be engaging in self-injurious behavior have been found to be lacking in verbal facility (Shodell & Reiter, 1968). *There appears to be a strong correlation between communication difficulties and the presence of problem behavior.*

This conceptualization is of particular contemporary importance because workers in this field are again proposing that behaviors such as aggression and self-injury may be similar to nonverbal forms of communication (e.g., Carr & Durand, 1985b; Day, Johnson, & Schussler, 1986; Donnellan et al., 1984; Durand, 1982, 1986b; Meyer & Evans, 1986; Neel et al.,

1983; Schuler & Goetz, 1981). It is useful here to discuss a context into which this work should be placed. It is just as necessary to outline what is not being suggested by analogies with communication, as it is to discuss the value of such a comparison.

In our work we have used *the concept of communication as a metaphor.* It has proven useful to compare challenging behavior to other forms of nonverbal behavior. The guidelines for assessment and intervention discussed here have all come from this comparison with communication. But, is problem behavior a form of communication? Problem behavior may have similarities with some definitions of communication, but it is impossible to make a definitive statement about its relationship to communication (Durand, 1986b). Thus, to date, we have avoided the conclusion that these behaviors *are* communication. Rather, conceptualizing challenging behavior in this way has been seen as being helpful in our intervention efforts.

Intervention Design

Many past and current efforts at designing interventions for behavior problems emphasize an *empirical approach.* Empirical, used in this context, refers to practices "guided by practical experience and not theory" (American Heritage Dictionary, 1973). This approach to intervention design relies on the use of a succession of procedures in a trial-and-error manner until one or more of these procedures effectively reduces the problem behavior. For example, if a student is biting his or her hand, intervention efforts might begin with attempts to ignore the biting. If hand biting was not reduced in a reasonable amount of time (e.g., 2 weeks), then a second intervention might be attempted (e.g., differential reinforcement of other behavior). Again, if this second intervention wasn't effective, then a third, fourth, and fifth intervention would be introduced in succession until one intervention was correlated with reduced hand biting. The guiding force behind decisions about which intervention to choose next typically involves going up a hierarchy of perceived restrictiveness or intrusiveness (i.e., from least to most restrictive or intrusive). There is no model or conceptualization of problem behavior that guides the clinical/educational decision-making process.

Although this tactic in intervention design has led to documented reductions in the problem behavior of many individuals, it is clear that the generalization and maintenance of such results have been limited (Durand & Carr, 1989; Harris & Ersner–Hershfield, 1978). It is conceivable that the failure of generalization and maintenance can, in part, be attributed to a lack of reliance on information about maintaining variables. For example, if a student is screaming to escape or avoid a boring task, it is possible that by contingently removing privileges, this screaming might be reduced. However, we might also expect other attempts to escape or avoid the tasks (e.g., through aggression, or getting up from his or her seat), and when the contingency is faded (but the task is not replaced) we would expect the student to resume screaming. *Without addressing why our students are misbehaving, the failure of our procedures to generalize to other persons or settings or to maintain over time should not be surprising.*

More recently, workers in this field have begun to incorporate information about the variables maintaining problem behavior into decisions regarding intervention. Thus, in contrast to the empirical approach, an increasing number of contemporary efforts emphasize a *prescriptive approach* to intervention design. The prescriptive approach combines the assessment of the functions of problem behavior with the design of interventions that address these functions. The intervention, then, is matched to the function of the behavior (Hayes, Nelson, & Jarrett, 1987). Therefore, what becomes of major interest to the clinician/educator is not *what* this person is doing (e.g., aggression or self-injury) but rather, *why* this person is doing it (e.g., to elicit attention or to avoid unpleasant tasks).

Using the previous example, a prescriptive approach to a student's screaming would first involve assessing that the behavior was in part maintained by the presence of the boring task. Intervention, therefore, might involve teaching him or her to request a new task or a break from work, and/or attempts to modify or perhaps even remove the troublesome task. In this book we adopt this prescriptive approach to intervention design.

In what follows, we will briefly review the research literature on the effectiveness of teaching alternate communicative (or other functionally equivalent) responses as a means of reducing problem behavior. Subsequent sections outline how we have translated this conceptualization into specific interventions. These studies represent the only experimental evidence for this hypothesis to date, and thus have both theoretical and educational implications. A growing number of studies have documented the effects of teaching functionally equivalent responses on the frequency of problem behavior, and these studies are described below.

Review of the Intervention Literature

Teaching functionally equivalent responses involves both the assessment of the function of the problem behavior and the teaching of a more appropriate form that serves the same function (e.g., verbal requests for attention). This type of intervention has been applied to severe forms of self-injurious behavior and aggression, as well as less dangerous behaviors, including stereotyped behavior and psychotic speech.

Dangerous Behavior

A number of studies have been conducted that demonstrate the value of this procedure in reducing severe behavior problems (e.g., Carr & Durand, 1985a; Durand, 1984; Durand & Carr, in press; Durand & Kishi, 1987; Horner & Budd, 1985; Smith, 1985; Smith & Coleman, 1986). In an early study, we worked with four adolescents and children who exhibited severe challenging behavior in the form of aggression, self-injurious behavior, and tantrums (Carr & Durand, 1985a). Analogue assessments were conducted to assess the role of easy and difficult tasks, as well as varying amounts of adult attention on these problem behaviors. The information gathered from these assessments suggested that both escape from academic demands and social attention may have been maintaining these students' problem behavior.

In order to rule out competing explanations, the interventions were conducted outside of the classroom, under highly controlled but artificial conditions. We found that if a student whose problem behavior was assessed as maintained by escape was taught to request social attention (through a phrase such as "Am I doing good work?"), there was no observed reduction in the problem behavior. However, if the same student was taught to request assistance on the task (through a phrase such as "I don't understand.") and received help by a teacher, then problem behavior was quickly reduced. Similarly, for students with problem behavior assessed to be maintained by social attention, teaching them to request assistance did not reduce problem behavior, but when they were taught to request attention and received it, their problem behaviors were reduced. This study demonstrated that teaching a functionally equivalent response could serve to replace and thus reduce the frequency of problem behavior.

Subsequent interventions have been conducted that further document the validity of this claim with a variety of other individuals and in a variety of other settings. In one example, we assessed the presumed function of the severe behavior problems of five adults with multiple handicaps (deaf and blind and severe/profound retardation) through the use of the Motivation Assessment Scale (Durand & Kishi, 1987). These adults were identified because they were engaging in severe and dangerous forms of aggression and self-injury. Based on the assessment information (i.e., that these behaviors were maintained by escape, social attention, and their tangible consequences), these individuals were taught to communicate requests nonverbally (through "tokens" with words written on them) that were equivalent to the assessed functions of their behavior problems (e.g., requests for assistance, requests for attention, and requests for tangibles). Intervention was conducted in both their residences (i.e., group homes, institution) and at their educational/vocational placements. This intervention resulted in significant improvements in the problem behavior of four of the adults at a 1-month follow-up visit. No change was observed in the behavior of one man, presumably because the staff did not continue training or respond to his requests. This study showed that communication training could be successful with persons who historically had difficulty with most communication training efforts.

Smith (1985) treated one 18-year-old man with autism who presumably engaged in aggression to obtain tangible reinforcers (i.e., food). Teaching him to request favorite foods verbally resulted in dramatic improvements in the number of his aggressive episodes. A similar study was conducted by Horner and Budd (1985). Unfortunately, because no formal assessment was conducted to determine the variables maintaining their student's problem behavior, interpreting this study as support for teaching functionally equivalent responses is problematic.

Bird, Dores, Moniz, and Robinson (1989) have recently documented the successful use of teaching functionally equivalent behavior with two adults with extensive histories of severe aggression and self-injury. Improvements were observed in problematic behavior as well as work productivity and the use of spontaneous communication, and these results were maintained over 6 months following intervention. This study is important because it documented that letting the men go on breaks from work did not result in decreased work productivity. This has been an area of concern for some caregivers (i.e., that the learners will stop participating in activities), but the data from Bird et al. (1989) do not support these misgivings.

Hunt, Alwell, and Goetz (1988) assessed the disruptive behaviors of three adolescents as possibly being maintained by peer attention. Participants in previous studies appeared to engage in problem behavior maintained by *adult* attention, thus making this study unique. The researchers found that when conversation skills with peers were taught, the disruptive behaviors of these high-school-aged individuals were significantly reduced. This study further documents the need to conduct a thorough analysis (e.g., differentiating the role of adult versus peer attention) prior to intervention.

Favell et al. (1982) worked with individuals engaging in self-injurious behavior maintained by sensory consequences. These researchers taught these individuals to manipulate toys that provided equivalent sensory input, and found that self-injurious behavior was substantially reduced. Thus, providing these individuals with a more appropriate way of obtaining their preferred reinforcers (i.e., through toy play rather than through self-injury) resulted in clinically significant improvements in these dangerous behaviors.

Stereotyped Behavior

A number of studies have found that teaching toy play can lead to reduced levels of stereotyped behavior (e.g., Azrin, Kaplan, & Foxx, 1973; Eason, White, & Newsom, 1982; Favell, 1973). A limitation of these studies is that there is no assessment of the function of the stereotyped behavior exhibited by the students. Thus, it is not clear that (1) these behaviors functioned to gain access to specific sensory input and, (2) that the types of toys these individuals were taught to play with provided alternative access to this sensory input. Research needs to be conducted that first uses an assessment methodology to determine the sensory function of these behaviors (e.g., sensory extinction) and second, demonstrates that teaching students to manipulate objects providing alternative sensory consequences will reduce stereotyped motor behavior. One example of this type of research (Rincover, Cook, Peoples, & Packard, 1979) demonstrated that for three of four students with autism, significant reductions in stereotyped behavior were observed during toy play that matched the function of their behavior. Additional work in this area is recommended to validate this type of treatment.

Some individuals appear to engage in stereotyped motor behavior for social reasons. For these individuals, then, functionally equivalent responses would include behavior that elicits specific social reactions by others (as opposed to producing specific sensory feedback). Following this reasoning, we assessed that the rocking and hand flapping of four individuals were maintained by escape from unpleasant situations (Durand & Carr, 1987). Using this information, these students were taught assistance-seeking responses (e.g., saying the phrase, "Help me") during difficult tasks. Figure 2-3 illustrates the effects of this intervention on rocking and hand flapping. This intervention resulted in significant reductions in stereotyped motor behavior for all four individuals. Although few studies have examined the efficacy of teaching functionally equivalent behavior as a treatment for stereotyped motor responses, this approach warrants further investigation given the nonaversive and constructive nature of this procedure.

Psychotic Speech

We recently applied the logic of teaching functionally equivalent behaviors, effectively applied with dangerous and stereotyped motor behavior, to the intervention of psychotic speech (Durand & Crimmins, 1987). The peculiar speech (phrases such as, "Parachute now" and "Fried eggs on your head") of one adolescent with autism appeared to be maintained by its ability to remove him from unpleasant situations. Therefore, he was taught to say "Help me" when faced with a difficult situation, in an effort to reduce the

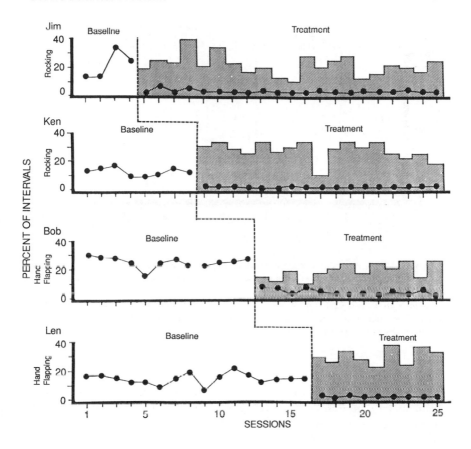

FIGURE 2-3. Percentage of intervals of stereotyped behavior during baseline and following communication training. The shaded areas represent the rate of the students' use of the phrase "Help me." From "Social Influences on 'Self-Stimulatory' Behavior: Analysis and Treatment Application" by V. M. Durand and E. G. Carr, 1987, *Journal of Applied Behavior Analysis, 20,* p. 128. Copyright 1987 by the Society for the Experimental Analysis of Behavior, Inc. Reprinted by permission of the authors and publisher.

unpleasantness of such things as academic tasks. This boy's data are presented in Figure 2-4. As can be seen in this graph, teaching him this functionally equivalent response (i.e., saying "Help me," which elicited trainer prompts which, in turn, presumably reduced the aversiveness of the training situation) resulted in significant reductions in psychotic speech at implementation, and moderately reduced levels at a 6-month follow-up. Thus, this socially mediated peculiar speech pattern was effectively treated by teaching an alternative assistance-seeking response. Similar results have been observed with echolalic speech among persons with autism (e.g.,

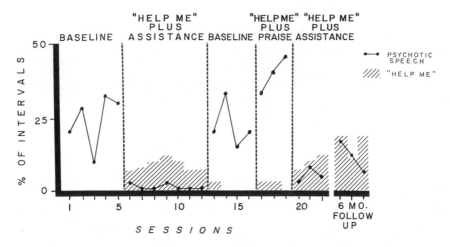

FIGURE 2-4. The percentage of intervals of psychotic speech and the student's use of the phrase "Help me" are presented during baseline, a control condition ("Help me" plus praise), and intervention ("Help me" plus assistance). From "Assessment and Treatment of Psychotic Speech in an Autistic Child" by V. M. Durand and D. B. Crimmins, 1987, *Journal of Autism and Developmental Disorders, 17*, p. 24. Copyright 1987 by Plenum Publishing Corporation. Reprinted by permission of the authors and publisher.

Schreibman & Carr, 1978). No equivalent research has been conducted on hallucinatory or delusional speech, although social functions have been hypothesized to play a part in the maintenance of these responses as well (Layng & Andronis, 1984).

Generalization and Maintenance

An important consideration in the evaluation of intervention effects is the assessment of generalization and maintenance. In other words, are the reductions in problem behavior observed during the initial intervention sessions carried over to other settings, with other persons, and across significant amounts of time? One criticism of aversive consequence-based interventions (e.g., time-out, contingent electric shock) has been that although they can often reduce the frequency of problem behavior initially, their effects are often temporary and/or limited to the intervention agent and setting in which intervention is conducted (e.g., Guess et al., 1987; Meyer & Evans, 1986; Murphy & Wilson, 1981). We have conducted two studies to determine whether or not generalization and maintenance occurs when teaching functionally equivalent responses.

In our first study in this series, we identified three boys who were reported to be extremely disruptive (e.g., they engaged highly frequent self-injury, aggression, and tantrums) in their classroom (Durand & Carr, in press). Assessments conducted with these students included analogue assessments as well as administrations of the MAS to their teacher. Functional communication training involved teaching all three boys to request assistance and, additionally, the third boy was also taught to request teacher attention appropriately. Extensive observational data collected in their classroom indicated that this intervention resulted in substantial improvements in their behavior.

Follow-up observations of the students in their new classrooms the following year indicated that two of the three students continued to use the phrases we taught them, and that they continued to engage in few problem behaviors. One student required additional work to articulate the trainer phrase so that his new teacher could understand it. Following this training, improvements in his problem behavior was again observed. A subsequent follow-up the next school year showed all three boys maintaining their improvements.

A second study was conducted to assess generalization further (Durand, 1984). Twelve students were selected for participation because they exhibited frequent problem behavior (e.g., aggression, self-injury, disruption), and because they were assessed to be engaging in these behaviors for adult attention. We compared functional communication training with the most widely used intervention for presumed attention-getting behavior, time-out from positive reinforcement. One group of 6 students received time-out (i.e., teacher stopped interacting with the student and turned away) when they exhibited an instance of problem behavior, and a second group of 6 was taught to elicit adult attention appropriately (i.e., through the use of a phrase such as, "Am I doing good work?"). Initial intervention for both groups was successful in significantly reducing their behavior problems.

Prior to intervention, we placed each student with a teacher who was naïve to our interventions, and monitored the students' behavior. We repeated this, following the students' participation in either the time-out intervention or functional communication training. We found that the time-out group resumed its disruptive behavior with the naïve teacher despite involvement in the previous intervention sessions. However, the group that received functional communication training did not resume its disruptive behavior with the teacher. It appears that this latter group "took its intervention with them." In other words, this group continued to request attention appropriately, and *without specific training*, the naïve teachers provided it. By providing this attention for verbal requests, these naïve teachers unknowingly reinforced a functionally equivalent response and thereby reduced disruptive behavior. In contrast, when the students in the time-out group were disruptive, many times the naïve teacher provided some form of attention (the teachers were not instructed on how to respond to problem behavior), thus reinforcing the continued presence of these behaviors.

One advantage of functional communication training may lie in its ability to be successful without specific training of others. As the previous studies indicated, without specific training and instruction, teachers will not carry out time-out procedures effectively with every student who is disruptive (nor should they!). Because this very specific intervention needs to be taught to everyone who may come in contact with the student, persons unfamiliar with the student or his or her program may inadvertently reinforce (thereby maintaining) instances of problem behavior. On the other hand, we did not have to teach teachers to respond to a verbal request for attention. When the students said, "Am I doing good work?" the teachers attended to them without instruction or prompts. The verbal requests allowed students to enter this "natural community of reinforcement" thereby maintaining their verbal requests and at the same time the reductions in their problem behaviors (Baer & Wolf, 1970).

Summary

The studies just reviewed suggest that significant improvements in the lives of persons with severe disabilities can be achieved through teaching functionally equivalent responses as a method of intervention for problem behavior. The introduction of any new technique should be viewed with caution, along with the initially optimistic results. However, given the replication of these results in a variety of settings and with a variety of research/clinical groups, there is room for optimism.

As noted above, one of the advantages of this method of intervention may lie not only in its ability to reduce problem behavior initially, but also in its ability to facilitate generalization and maintenance of treatment gains (Durand, 1987; Horner & Billingsley, 1988). Because our technology for teaching adaptive responses that generalize and maintain well over time is quite advanced when compared to our behavior reduction technology, this should allow us to provide more lasting and durable interventions (Stokes & Baer, 1977). Successful generalization and maintenance of functionally equivalent responses should, in turn, lead to generalization and maintenance of reductions in problem behavior. What follows is a discussion of the assessment process we follow in preparation for functional communication training.

3

Assessment

With Daniel B. Crimmins

"In order to find anything—you must be looking for something."
(VARELA, 1977, p. 921)

Virtually all professionals feel that some type of assessment is necessary before an intervention for severe problem behavior should begin. Although there is a high level of agreement that assessment should occur, there is not a corresponding level of agreement as to *how* this should occur. Clearly, the desirable outcome from an assessment procedure is an intervention plan with a good chance for success. This chapter will discuss assessment procedures with the intent of assisting the reader in achieving more desirable intervention results.

Jonathan

Jonathan is an 8-year-old boy who has been diagnosed as having autism. Jonathan's teacher requested help in dealing with his problem behaviors because she finds them to be particularly disruptive. His teacher reports that he is belligerent and oppositional, and that this occurs constantly throughout the day. She suggested that this negative behavior was probably due to being abandoned by his parents at the age of 6 months, and that the anger was building up inside of him. She also noted that he does not seem to like any of the reinforcers they try to give him in the classroom, often pushing them away. Previous attempts to reduce these oppositional behaviors through various means (for example, trying to get him to express his anger, reinforcing him for not being oppositional, and time-out) all proved to be unsuccess-

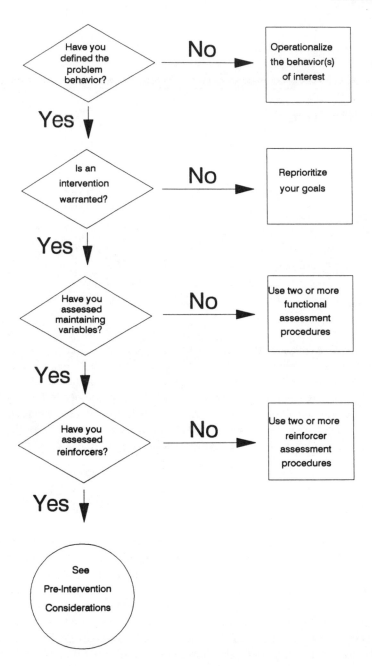

FIGURE 3-1. The assessment process.

ful. The teacher working with Jonathan was thoroughly frustrated with him, and was looking for an alternative placement.

This all-too-familiar story illustrates a number of important assessment issues that we will address in this section. First, just what was Jonathan doing that was making his teacher so upset? Being "belligerent" and "oppositional" could simply mean that he does not comply with all of his teacher's requests, or it could mean that he hits others and/or himself when asked to do the most basic tasks. It is extremely important to be able to describe clearly the actual behaviors engaged in by the student. Second, do you design an intervention for this problem? Who decides whether or not to intervene, and how should you decide this? Third, how do you assess for those variables that may be contributing to the continued presence of problem behaviors? Do you look for past incidents that may influence current behavior (e.g., being abandoned at 6 months), or are contemporary influences more important (e.g., just being asked to do something he didn't want to do)? This assessment is obviously important, but just how should you go about collecting this information? And, what do you do with this information once you collect it? Fourth, all too often, teachers are not successful in identifying powerful reinforcers for their students. How should you select reinforcers? The answers to these general questions will be covered in this section on assessment. Figure 3-1 illustrates the assessment steps we follow in this chapter. Each aspect will be described in some detail.

Defining Problem Behavior

This step is probably the most obvious, and is also one of the more over-looked aspects of assessment. It should become clear that as we talk about a behavior's "function" (in other words, why this student is behaving this way), specifying the behavior or behaviors that are a problem becomes extremely important. Using the example of Jonathan illustrated above, describing his behavior as being belligerent or oppositional does not give you a complete picture. Does he scream and cry when he doesn't want to do things? Does he bite his hand or attempt to hit others? Is he just passively resistant? Suppose, for example, that he occasionally does engage in each of these behaviors (screaming, crying, hand biting, hitting others, and no response to commands). However, let us further suppose that he screams and cries when he wants your attention, that he bites his hand and hits you when you take away a favorite toy, and that he resists passively when he doesn't want to work. This suggests that each of these behaviors may need *different interventions*. Ignoring screaming and crying may be a good approach because he wants to get your attention with these behaviors. Yet, ignoring

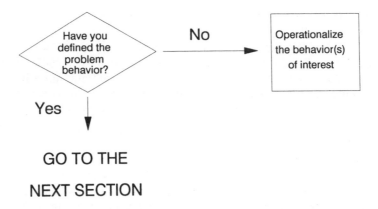

(that is, walking away from) his passive resistance may actually make it increase because it may get him what he wants (the end of work).

The example above should illustrate the danger of combining too many behaviors into general catagories such as "tantrums," "opposition," or "disruption." It is extremely important that the separate behaviors a student engages in are identified, and attempts are made to assess their separate influences. This should be done through *operational definitions*; descriptions of behaviors that are *observable* and *measurable* (Sulzer–Azaroff & Reese, 1982). The guiding principle here is that the behavior(s) should be described in such as way that a person who may never have observed the student would nonetheless easily recognize these responses. For example, as we saw above, "belligerence" may be seen as different things to different persons. "Hand biting," however, is something we can all see and could measure (in other words, we could count the number of times a student put his teeth on his hand). Below are some examples of good descriptions and poor descriptions of behaviors.

Poor	*Good*
Tantrums	Screaming
Disruption	Falling on the floor
Self-abuse	Face slapping
Aggression	Pinching others
Assaultive	Pushing others

Again, the emphasis on this point is important because it has direct implications for later intervention efforts. Not only will it be difficult to communicate to others if you do not have a good description of the behavior of interest, you may also be grouping together behaviors that may need separate interventions.

Should You Intervene?

Clearly, a decision that needs to be made prior to intervention is whether or not an intervention is necessary. Evans and Meyer (1985) meticulously describe issues related to selecting behaviors to target for intervention, and readers are directed to this excellent book for a detailed discussion (for additional perspectives, see Gaylord—Ross, 1980; Hawkins, 1986; Renzaglia & Bates, 1983; Sulzer—Azaroff & Reese, 1982; Tharp & Wetzel, 1969). Voeltz, Evans, Freedland, and Donellon (1982) identified six major groups of concerns that were identified by special education teachers and PhD students as important for intervention consideration: "urgent child need," "concern for others," "child's adjustment," "positive repertoire," "functional for the child," "instructional utility." Evans and Meyer have taken these concerns and translated them into a series of specific issues. We have summarized many of the issues raised by Evans and Meyer into a series of questions asked of parents, teachers, and others, and these are described in Figures 3-2 and 3-3.

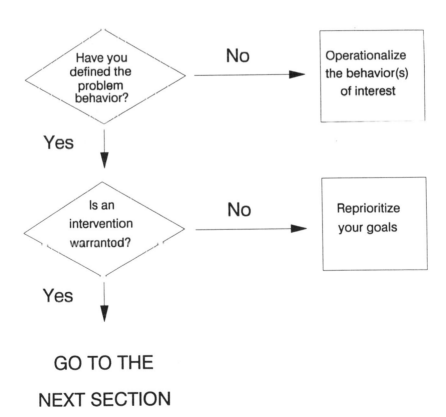

SUBJECTIVE ASSESSMENT OF PROBLEM BEHAVIOR SCALE

Student's Name: _Jonathan_   Date: _7/11/89_
Rater's Name: _Wendy_   Location of Rating: _Home_

Rater's Title: _Mother_

Identified Problem Behavior: _Screaming_

1. Is this behavior life-threatening?   YES   (NO)

2. Does this behavior provide a health   YES   (NO)
   risk to the student?

3. Does this behavior interfere with   (YES)   NO
   learning?

4. Is this behavior likely to become   (YES)   NO
   serious in the near future if not
   modified?

5. Is this behavior dangerous to   YES   (NO)
   others?

6. Is this behavior of great concern   (YES)   NO
   to caregivers?

7. Is this behavior getting worse or   YES   (NO)
   not improving?

8. Has this been a problem for some   YES   (NO)
   time?

9. Does this behavior damage materials?   YES   (NO)

10. Does this behavior interfere with   (YES)   NO
    community acceptance?

11. Would other behaviors improve if   (YES)   NO
    this behavior improved?

FIGURE 3-2. Hypothetical data on Jonathan's screaming. From *An Educative Approach to Behavior Problems* by I. M. Evans and L. H. Meyer, 1985, Baltimore: Paul H. Brookes. Copyright 1985 by Paul H. Brookes, Inc. Adapted by permission of the authors and publisher.

SUBJECTIVE ASSESSMENT OF PROBLEM BEHAVIOR SCALE

Student's Name: __Jonathan__   Date: __7/11/89__
Rater's Name: __WENDY__   Location of Rating: __HOME__

Rater's Title: __MOTHER__

Identified Problem Behavior: __HAND BITING__

---

1. Is this behavior life-threatening?	YES	(NO)
2. Does this behavior provide a health risk to the student?	(YES)	NO
3. Does this behavior interfere with learning?	(YES)	NO
4. Is this behavior likely to become serious in the near future if not modified?	(YES)	NO
5. Is this behavior dangerous to others?	YES	(NO)
6. Is this behavior of great concern to caregivers?	(YES)	NO
7. Is this behavior getting worse or not improving?	(YES)	NO
8. Has this been a problem for some time?	(YES)	NO
9. Does this behavior damage materials?	YES	(NO)
10. Does this behavior interfere with community acceptance?	(YES)	NO
11. Would other behaviors improve if this behavior improved?	(YES)	NO

FIGURE 3-3. Hypothetical data on Jonathan's hand biting. From *An Educative Approach to Behavior Problems* by I. M. Evans and L. H. Meyer, 1985, Baltimore: Paul H. Brookes. Copyright 1985 by Paul H. Brookes, Inc. Adapted by permission of the authors and publisher.

These scales show how Jonathan's mother responded for his hand biting and screaming. As can be seen from her answers, both behaviors interfere with learning and community acceptance, and both are of concern. However, in addition, hand biting poses a health risk and has been a problem for some time. It would be recommended that hand biting be targeted first for assessment and intervention. If screaming was not also reduced following the intervention, then it would be addressed next.

We routinely request that parents, teachers, and/or other staff answer the questions presented in this scale prior to designing an intervention. As we have seen, this is especially important if decisions need to be made as to which of several problem behaviors require a program. It is not uncommon for teachers or parents to identify an extensive list of disruptive behaviors displayed by a student. One way to distinguish among behaviors to target is to estimate their effect on the person exhibiting the behavior (e.g., "Is this behavior life threatening?") or on others (e.g., "Is this behavior dangerous to others?").

In addition to the concerns outlined above, other considerations are necessary prior to designing an intervention. For example, we have observed times when the "problem" really belongs to the staff, teacher, or even the program the student is attending. There may be times when it is *our* behavior that should be changed, and not the behavior of those with whom we work. For example, a director of a work project once asked for consultation concerning a woman who was working in his program. The problem he described was that the woman would frequently leave the work site and would occasionally run out of the building and into the street. The director was fearful that someday she would be seriously hurt by a passing car. Upon further examination, it was mentioned that she worked in the kitchen, and that the real problem was with washing dishes. She would become upset if she had to wash dishes and would sometimes run outside. The director was requesting an incentive program to help keep her on the job.

In an attempt to provide the director with a different perspective, he was asked what he would do if he was in a job that he really didn't like. Without hesitation, he said he would quit. It was then suggested that he let this woman quit, and find another job. She should probably be taught a better way to express her displeasure with assigned tasks, but it was reasonable for her not to like every job provided. The director explained that this was the only job available in his program. Fortunately, further questioning brought out that she seemed to enjoy the other jobs in the kitchen (e.g., cleaning the floor, drying and putting away the dishes), and that she didn't run away from them. It was recommended that she be assigned only to these other tasks, and that communication training be initiated to get her to request reassignments appropriately.

The main point of this example is that many programs that provide services to persons with developmental disabilities at times lose perspective on the nature of their goals. Is the goal to teach participants, for example, to work at and like every job, or is it to provide opportunities for employment (or play, relationships, education, etc.) that allow for matches of preference and ability? Often, the issue of "person—environment fit" is lost in the practicalities of running a program (Schalock, Harper, & Genung, 1981). The issue raised by the previous example is that there are times when the "problem" lies in the system created, and not in the people being served.

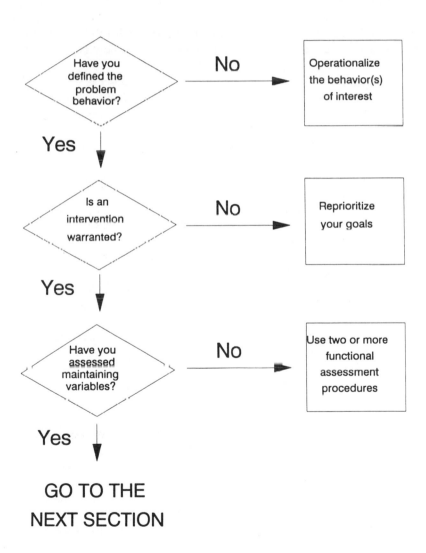

Assessing Influences on Problem Behavior

To paraphrase a quote on psychotherapy by Gordon Paul (1967), an essential question to answer for assessment is "Why is *this* person engaging in *this* behavior, in *this* setting, at *this* time?" Assessment procedures for a severe problem behavior can focus on many aspects of this question. And, although a variety of procedures are in wide use, we have identified a number of different, and potentially related, outcomes of typical assessment procedures. First, for example, an assessment might provide a description of the frequency and topography of the behavior. Second, it might attempt to define conditions in which the behavior is more likely to occur. Third, assessment might identify those events that typically follow a behavior's occurrence and might constitute a class of variables that are likely to be maintaining the behavior—that is, serving as reinforcers for it.

Secondary questions surrounding the assessment process relate to why one is assessing the behavior now and how that information will be used. Too often, assessment is conducted without a thoughtful response to these questions, and at times, interventions are begun before any assessment is conducted. Procedures for assessment are not necessarily based only in the present. Typically, we also seek historical information about a behavior. For example, it is often useful to know about other attempts to reduce the frequency of a problem behavior before designing an intervention plan. Questions that might be asked include: Were they successful and for how long? Why were they stopped? Why did they fail? What alternative behaviors were taught? Did the individual use those behaviors?

Assessment of problem behaviors should lead to development of a plan on how to respond to them. It is suggested throughout this book that assessment information should guide decision making about the selection of the best possible intervention strategy that is likely to be successful with a specific behavior problem. *In our experience, assessment too often consists of only counting behaviors;* frequency is one method of describing the impact of a behavior on the others in the environment. However, knowing the frequency rarely leads to a plan. In situations where a clinician/educator already has an intervention selected for a particular behavior, counting the occurrences (or recording the duration) of the behavior to establish a baseline may provide a comparison to postintervention rates of the behavior that allows a judgment as to the intervention's effectiveness. We acknowledge that it is important to have data of this type to support claims of intervention effectiveness. However, the use of data for evaluation and for assessment should be seen as independent.

Almost every writer on the subject of severe behavior problems has warned clinicians, educators, and other service providers that, prior to implementing any intervention, an effort should be made to assess for the variables controlling these behaviors. Attempting a functional analysis has been seen as important because intervention may be unsuccessful if the variables maintaining the targeted behavior are not identified and the learner is not provided with an alternative means of obtaining these reinforcers. Until recently, however, there have been few specific guidelines for conducting a functional analysis (Voeltz, Evans, Derer, & Hanashiro, 1983). In this section we will review a variety of different assessment methodologies that are designed for gathering information about severe behavior problems. Specifically, the goal of these assessments is to generate hypotheses as to the variables maintaining these behaviors. Reviewed together will be methods designed to assess stimulus events and setting events. Information on assessing setting events will necessarily be brief because of the limited assessment research in this area.

An Overview

Figure 3-4 illustrates one way of viewing current efforts at assessing the influences on problem behavior. We have divided the varying ways of collecting this information into (1) when the information is gathered (i.e., retrospectively or concurrently with the behavior problem), and (2) the status of the prevailing environment (i.e., whether it remains intact or is modified). For example, observing a student in a classroom for any patterns that might predict problem behavior would be concurrent information (collected at the time the behavior problem occurs) in an intact environment (no changes are made in the student's daily routine). On the other hand, reviewing the student's records for the effects of previous interventions would be an example of retrospective collection of information (gathered from past information) from a modified environment (the interventions represent planned changes in the environment). We use this overview to review assessment methods below.

What follows is a review of the assessment methods currently being used to collect information on the variables maintaining problem behavior. Table 3-1 lists these methods, and summarizes the advantages and disadvantages of each approach. It is important to note here that *no single assessment methodology is recommended*. It is always best if converging information about these variables can be obtained. In other words if, for example, direct "naturalistic" observations about a behavior reveal the same information as a rating scale, then we would have more confidence in that information. All forms of assessment include sources of error (including direct observation). Therefore, we never can be completely certain of the variables maintaining problem behavior. Yet, our hypotheses are better if two or more methods agree. Readers interested in more detailed information

STATE OF THE ENVIRONMENT

INFORMATION GATHERING	Intact	Modified
Retrospective	Clinical intuition Structured interviews Rating scales	Record reviews Logs/Incident reports
Concurrent	Informal observations Scatter plots "ABC" charts Setting event checklist	Analogue assessments

FIGURE 3-4. A conceptual overview of the types of assessment methods used to assess the function of challenging behavior.

should refer to more extensive discussion on this topic elsewhere (e.g., Anastasi, 1982; Cronbach, Gleser, Nanda, & Rajaratnam, 1972; Haynes & Horn, 1982; Nelson & Hayes, 1986).

Retrospective Information from Intact Environments

CLINICAL INTUITION

Perhaps the most common method of assessing the variables maintaining problem behavior is *guessing*. Guessing (or clinical intuition) typically occurs at an interdisciplinary team meeting where several persons familiar with the student in question hypothesize about the relative influence of numerous variables based solely on their usually unsystematic recollections. Characteristically, the hypothesis adopted is related more to the persuasiveness of the speaker than its relationship to reality. Our data suggest that guessing, even by teachers with extensive histories with their students, is not predictive of how these students will later behave (Durand & Crimmins, 1988).

TABLE 3-1. Assessment methods

Procedure	Example	Advantages	Disadvantages
Clinical intuition		Possibility of sampling a wide range of stimuli Ease of Use	Lacks demonstrated reliability and validity No specific guidelines to assist identifying stimuli Retrospective reporting of events
Structured interviews	Bailey & Pyles, 1989 O'Neil et al., 1989	Possibility of sampling a wide range of stimuli Ease of use Specific guidelines to assist in identifying stimuli	Retrospective reporting of events Lack reliability and validity
Rating scales	Durand & Crimmins, 1988 Wiesler et al., 1985	Ease of use Some have demonstrated reliability and validity Specific guidelines to assist in identifying stimuli	Some scales lack demonstrated reliability and validity Retrospective reporting of events
Record reviews	Crimmins & Durand, in press	Can assess history of successes and failures Ease of use	Sample of stimuli limited to history of assessment and intervention and to thoroughness of documentation Lack of reliability and validity No specific guidelines to assist in identifying stimuli Retrospective reporting of events
Informal observations	Repp et al., 1988	Possibility of sampling a wide range of stimuli Ease of use	Lack of reliability and validity No specific guidelines to assist in identifying stimuli
Logs/Incident reports	Meyer & Evans, 1989	Ease of use Some provide guidelines to assist in identifying stimuli Concurrent reporting of events	Lack reliability and validity Sample of stimuli assessed guided by form used and training of staff
Scatter plot	Touchette et al., 1985	Ease of use Can point to schedule and activity related influences Concurrent reporting of events	Limited guidelines for assessing stimuli Limited validity data

(cont.)

TABLE 3-1 (cont.)

Procedure	Example	Advantages	Disadvantages
Formal observations	Bijou et al., 1968 Evans & Meyers, 1985	Ease of use Possibility of sampling a wide range of stimuli Concurrent reporting of events	Limited guidelines for assessing stimuli Lack of reliability and validity
Analogue Assessments	Durand & Crimmins, 1988 Iwata et al., 1982	Possibility of sampling a wide range of stimuli Concurrent reporting of events Experimental demonstration of influence	Difficult to conduct in some settings Can be time consuming and labor intensive Limited use with life-threatening behavior

Clinical intuition is mentioned here as a caveat. It *is* important to get information from those who know the students best. And historical information (e.g., how they misbehaved in the past and under what circumstances) is also invaluable. However, because more formal methods of collecting this information exist (some of which have demonstrated reliability and validity), it is recommended that those involved with the decision-making process look to these additional, and perhaps more valid methods, for assessing behavior problems.

STRUCTURED INTERVIEWS

One method that has recently been proposed as an additional method for assessing past instances of behavior problems is the use of structured interviews (e.g., Bailey & Pyles, 1989; O'Neill, Horner, Albin, Storey, & Sprague, 1989). For example, the interview described by O'Neill and colleagues involves questioning teachers, parents, and any other concerned persons about the nature of the behavior problem(s) and possible controlling variables. Questions concern the respective roles of such things as medication, sleep, eating routines, and daily activities on the behaviors of interest. This approach has advantages over less formal questioning because of the structured nature of the questions. Because a variety of influences are surveyed each time and with each individual, important influences are less likely to be overlooked.

An important limitation of the proposed structured interviews that is common to most of the assessment strategies reviewed here is that there is no demonstrated reliability or validity. For example, would the same answers and conclusions be made if two individuals were interviewed separately (e.g., a teacher and an aide)? Will the conclusions made from the interview predict how the student will behave later (e.g., scream if a toy is taken away)? Such interviews *may* be reliable and valid, but to date there have been no such demonstrations. Therefore, persons using such interviews should be cautious about the conclusions drawn from them. Again, one safeguard is to use *multiple* forms of assessment to strengthen the inferences made about why a student is misbehaving.

RATING SCALES

Behavior rating scales have existed for years, often focusing on whether an individual displays specific topographies of problem behaviors. They are, in fact, often incorporated into routine assessments of adaptive behavior. The Vineland Adaptive Behavior Scales (Sparrow, Balla, & Cicchetti, 1984), for example, seek information on 36 different types of behavior. This is one of many such scales that focus on the whether or not an individual engages in a specific problem behavior. However, these scales do not consider the functional significance of the behavior.

More recently rating scales have been developed that attempt to address the issue of the function of problem behavior. In an effort to provide an alternative assessment method, several authors have developed rating scales (e.g., Donnellan et al., 1984; Durand & Crimmins, 1983,1988; Schuler, Peck, Tomlinson, & Theimer, 1984; Wieseler, Hanson, Chamberlain, & Thompson, 1985). These scales are designed to be completed by caregivers, and ask questions about the variables that may be maintaining challenging behavior. The scales vary in terms of ease of use and the degree to which the findings can lead to the development of an intervention plan. Described here will be the Motivation Assessment Scale (MAS; Durand, 1988; Durand & Crimmins, 1983, 1988), because it is currently the only scale of this kind with demonstrated reliability and validity. Because its use has been integral to developing plans with functional communication training, we will discuss the use of the MAS in some detail. It should be noted that the MAS is typically used early in the assessment process. As will be seen in the next section, the results of this scale can then be used to guide further assessment efforts or to develop a preliminary intervention plan.

THE MOTIVATION ASSESSMENT SCALE

The MAS was developed over a period of several years with the help of numerous teachers, parents, and service providers of persons with autism and other developmental disabilities. During the years, numerous questions were added and deleted from the scale. Questions and wordings were tested until it became clear that persons involved in the care of individuals with developmental disabilities could, through the scale, adequately report how these individuals would behave in situations such as difficult tasks, unstructured settings, being denied reinforcers, and in settings with reduced adult attention. The resulting scale is a 16-item questionnaire that assesses the functional significance of behavior (see Figure 3-5) along the dimensions of sensory, escape/avoidance, social attention, and tangible rewards.

Administration of the MAS. Individuals filling out the MAS may be parents, teachers, or other individuals who have had close contact with the person exhibiting the problem behavior. The raters are asked to circle the number estimating the probability of the target behavior occurring in each of the 16 situations (see example in Figure 3-5). Recall that these conditions are organized into four motivational classes (attention, tangible, escape, and sensory), with four questions for each class.

Specifying the Target Behavior. We have found it important to re-emphasize to raters using the MAS the need to *select a specific behavior (e.g., hits his head) rather than a more general description of the individual's behavior (e.g., get's upset).* Often raters select a behavioral definition that is too broad and end up scoring several behaviors that may be maintained by different variables. For example, one girl's tantrum may, in different settings, include such behaviors as hand biting, screaming, and running around the room. However, hand biting and screaming may be used to escape demanding situations, although running around the room may be used in other situations to gain attention. Therefore, rating these behaviors together as a "tantrum" may result in results that are difficult to interpret. Care must be taken to identify different topographies of problem behavior, and have raters assess these behaviors separately. Because the MAS takes from 5 to 10 minutes to complete, completing separate scales for each of several behavior problems is not a difficult task.

Specifying the Setting. In addition to specifying the individual behavior problems, it is also important that raters assess these behaviors for different settings. The importance of this is easily underscored in educational settings where students might receive speech therapy in a one-to-one setting, adaptive physical education in a group setting, and be exposed to a variety of instructional groupings in the classroom. In the general setting of "the school" there can, therefore, be a number of different settings that might best be considered separately. Again, because of its ease of use, *it is recommended that the MAS be filled out separately for each setting in which the behavior is a problem.*

Scoring. Scoring the MAS is relatively simple. The number circled for each question is entered on the blank next to the question number on the back of the form. Each column of numbers is totaled separately and a mean (total/4) is calculated. The first column mean corresponds to the score for sensory consequences as the maintaining variable, the second column for escape from unpleasant situations, the third for social attention, and the fourth for tangible consequences. As you can see from the example MAS completed for "Jim," his *hand biting* in *articulation training sessions* is most likely to be maintained by escape from unpleasant situations. Ranked number two was tangible consequences, number three was attention, and number four was sensory consequences.

Interpreting the MAS. Proper scoring of the MAS typically yields the identification of one or more variables that may be maintaining a student's problem behavior. If one category of maintaining variables has clearly received the highest score, then it is assumed that this has the most important influence on this behavior. If several categories are given high scores and are nearly identical (e.g., within a mean of .25 to .50 points), then they may all be important influences. In the case of multiple influences, it is often helpful to specify further the setting in which you may be concerned about the student's behavior. For example, one MAS could be filled out for hand biting during seat work, although a second MAS could be completed for hand biting in group instruction. It is often the case that by further specifying settings or behaviors, one influence stands out as dominant in that circumstance. The variable with the highest mean score (e.g., escape) is assumed to be an important maintaining variable for the *specified behavior* in the *specified setting.* As noted in the example above, Jim's hand biting during articulation training sessions appears to be maintained by escape from unpleasant situations.

Research. Durand and Crimmins (1988) describe the first data on reliability and validity for the MAS. The reliability study was conducted with the teachers of 50 students with developmental disabilities who exhibited self-injurious behavior. These students came from four states, ranged in age from 3 to 18, and had received diagnoses that included severe mental retardation and autism. Interrater reliability (i.e., data from the student's teacher and assistant teacher) was measured by Pearson correlation coefficients, and ranged from .80 to .95. Test–retest reliability (i.e., data from the teachers' MAS responses 30 days apart) was also measured by Pearson correlation coefficients, and ranged from .89 to .98. These data suggest that the MAS is a reliable instrument. Two raters can generally agree on the variables maintaining a student's problem behavior, and this rating remains stable over time.

Name __JIM__ Rater __WENDY__ Date __6/4/89__

Behavior Description __HAND BITING - anytime Jim's teeth touch__
__his hands in a forceful manner (i.e., it leaves a mark or cut)__

Setting Description __articulation training__

Instructions: The **Motivation Assessment Scale** is a questionnaire designed to identify those situations in which an individual is likely to behave in certain ways. From this information, more informed decisions can be made concerning the selection of appropriate reinforcers and treatments. To complete the **Motivation Assessment Scale**, select one behavior that is of particular interest. It is important that you identify the behavior *very specifically.* *Aggressive,* for example, is not as good a description as *hits his sister.* Once you have specified the behavior to be rated, reac each question carefully and circle the *one* number that best describes your observations of this behavior.

ANSWERS

QUESTIONS

	Never	Almost Never	Seldom	Half the Time	Usually	Almost Always	Always
1. Would the behavior occur continuously, over and over, if this person was left alone for long periods of time? (For example, several hours.)	0	(1)	2	3	4	5	6
2. Does the behavior occur following a request to perform a difficult task?	0	1	2	3	4	(5)	6
3. Does the behavior seem to occur in response to your talking to other persons in the room?	0	1	(2)	3	4	5	6
4. Does the behavior ever occur to get a toy, food, or activity that this person has been told that he or she can't have?	0	1	2	(3)	4	5	6

48

	Never 0	Almost Never 1	Seldom 2	Half the Time 3	Usually 4	Almost Always 5	Always 6

5. Would the behavior occur repeatedly, in the same way, for very long periods of time, if no one was around? (For example, rocking back and forth for over an hour?)
— Almost Never (1)

6. Does the behavior occur when *any* request is made of this person?
— Usually (4)

7. Does the behavior occur whenever you stop attending to this person?
— Almost Never (1)

8. Does the behavior occur when you take away a favorite toy, food, or activity?
— Half the Time (3)

9. Does it appear to you that this person enjoys performing the behavior? (It feels, tastes, looks, smells, and/or sounds pleasing.)
— Never (0)

10. Does this person seem to do the behavior to upset or annoy you when you are trying to get him or her to do what you ask?
— Almost Always (5)

11. Does this person seem to do the behavior to upset or annoy you when you are not paying attention to him or her? (For example, if you are sitting in a separate room interacting with another person.)
— Never (0)

12. Does the behavior **stop** occurring shortly after you give this person the toy, food or activity he or she has requested?
— Half the Time (3)

13. When the behavior is occurring, does this person seem calm and unaware of anything else going on around him or her?
— Almost Never (1)

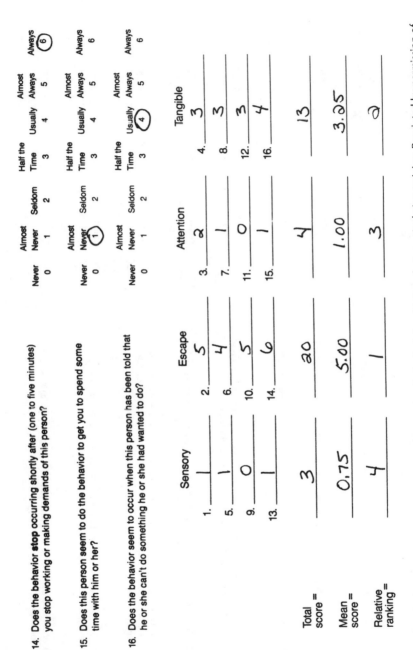

14. Does the behavior **stop** occurring shortly after (one to five minutes) you stop working or making demands of this person?

| Never 0 | Almost Never 1 | Seldom 2 | Half the Time 3 | Usually 4 | Almost Always 5 | Always (6) |

15. Does this person seem to do the behavior to **get** you to spend some time with him or her?

| Never 0 | Almost Never (1) | Seldom 2 | Half the Time 3 | Usually 4 | Almost Always 5 | Always 6 |

16. Does the behavior seem to occur when this person has been told that he or she can't do something he or she had wanted to do?

| Never 0 | Almost Never 1 | Seldom 2 | Half the Time 3 | Usually (4) | Almost Always 5 | Always 6 |

Sensory	Escape	Attention	Tangible
1. 3	2. 5	3. 2	4. 3
5. 1	6. 4	7. 1	8. 3
9. 0	10. 5	11. 0	12. 3
13. 1	14. 6	15. 1	16. 4
Total score = 3	20	4	13
Mean score = 0.75	5.00	1.00	3.25
Relative ranking = 4	1	3	2

FIGURE 3-5. A completed Motivation Assessment Scale for Jim's hand biting during articulation training. Reprinted by permission of V. Mark Durand, State University of New York at Albany.

The second study compared teacher's ratings on the MAS with the student's behavior in a variety of analogue assessment conditions. Figures 3-6 through 3-9 show the data on self-injurious behavior for eight students. Figure 3-6 represents the results from the analogue conditions for two students rated on the MAS by their teachers as having "attention-getting" self-injury. This graph shows that most of the students' self-injurious behavior occurred when social attention was reduced (Attention condition). Similarly, Figure 3-7 illustrates the data from two students with self-injury rated as "escape-maintained." Their self-injury occurred most often when tasks were more difficult (Escape condition). Figure 3-8 represents data from students rated as having "tangibly maintained" self-injury, and their behavior problems occurred most often when favorite tangibles were available at reduced levels (Tangible condition). Finally, Figure 3-9 shows graphs of data for two students rated as having "sensory-maintained" behavior problems. Their self-injury was most likely to occur when attention was available, tasks were present but they were not prompted to work, and favorite tangibles were available (Unstructured condition).

All of the rating on the MASs and all of the analogue conditions were conducted anonymously. Neither the teachers filling out the scales, nor the experimenters running the assessment sessions knew of the others' results. These data support the validity of the MAS, because *the teachers' ratings on the scale predicted how the students would behave in analogue settings.* It should be noted that the students in this study were engaging in self-injury that was moderately frequent (mean greater than 15 instances per hour). When assessing behaviors occurring much more frequently (e.g., more than 15 per minute) or much less frequently (e.g., less than once per day), care should be taken if using the MAS, because reliability and validity data have not been established for these extremes.

WHY NOT JUST ASK CAREGIVERS?

One question that is often asked when discussing the MAS has to do with its necessity. Would simply asking teachers, parents, or others if a student's problem behavior was maintained by attention, escape, tangibles, or sensory consequences yield the same information as a full administration of the scale? In order to answer this question, we asked the teachers in the previous study to rank the four classes of maintaining variables for their possible influence on the students' self-injurious behaviors. We observed that these rankings did not correlate significantly with the teachers' MAS scores. Therefore, *although teachers could predict their students' self-injurious behavior through their answers on the MAS, their global ratings of controlling variables were not as accurate.*

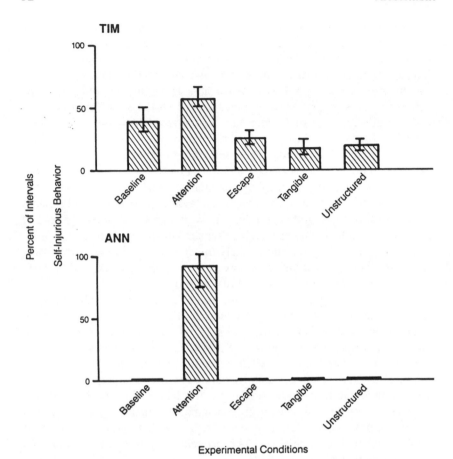

FIGURE 3-6. The percentage of self-injurious behavior in each experimental condition exhibited by the two students (Tim and Ann) rated as having "attention-getting" self-injury on the MAS. From "Identifying the Variables Maintaining Self-Injurious Behavior" by V. M. Durand and D. B. Crimmins, 1988, *Journal of Autism and Developmental Disorders, 18,* pp. 110–113. Copyright 1988 by Plenum Publishing Corporation. Reprinted by permission of the authors and publisher.

EXTREMELY HIGH FREQUENCY BEHAVIOR

For some individuals, problem behavior can be exhibited so frequently so as to make a functional analysis almost impossible. For example, one woman we worked with engaged in head hitting at a rate exceeding 175 times per minute. With this woman's self-injury, we did not observe changes in frequency in different settings, partly because we couldn't let her hit herself

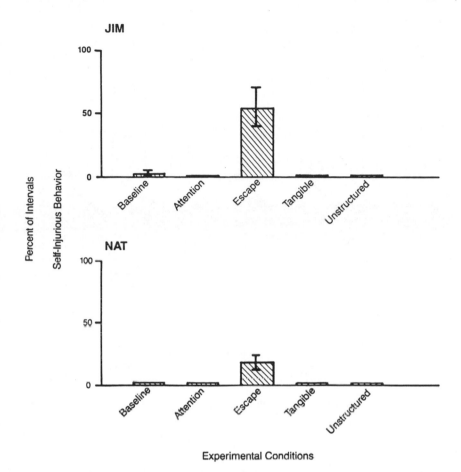

FIGURE 3-7. The percentage of self-injurious behavior in each experimental condition exhibited by the two students (Jim and Nat) rated as having "escape-maintained" self-injury on the MAS. From "Identifying the Variables Maintaining Self-Injurious Behavior" by V. M. Durand and D. B. Crimmins, 1988, *Journal of Autism and Developemntal Disorders, 18,* pp. 110–113. Copyright 1988 by Plenum Publishing Corporation. Reprinted by permission of the authors and publisher.

too many times and risk serious injury. However, when we asked staff to rate just "hard hits" on the MAS (and not her light "taps"), we observed reliable reports of the possible controlling variables (in this case, escape). In those instances where there are behaviors occurring almost constantly, it may be useful to delineate further the behaviors by such factors as intensity (e.g., hard and soft hits).

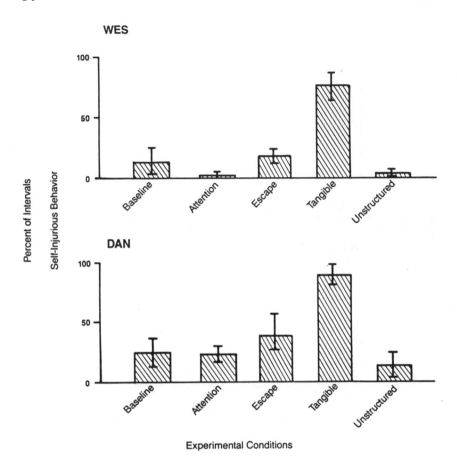

FIGURE 3-8. The percentage of self-injurious behavior in each experimental condition exhibited by the two students (Wes and Dan) rated as having "tangibly maintained" self-injury on the MAS. From "Identifying the Variables Maintaining Self-Injurious Behavior" by V. M. Durand and D. B. Crimmins, 1988, *Journal of Autism and Developemntal Disorders, 18,* pp. 110–113. Copyright 1988 by Plenum Publishing Corporation. Reprinted by permission of the authors and publisher.

EXTREMELY LOW FREQUENCY BEHAVIOR

Behaviors that occur less than once per day, week or month can be extremely difficult to assess. Although we have used the MAS with these behaviors to provide some information, we have also attempted to use several other forms of assessment (e.g., analogues). Especially in situations where you may doubt the validity of your information, collecting information from a variety of sources is most valuable.

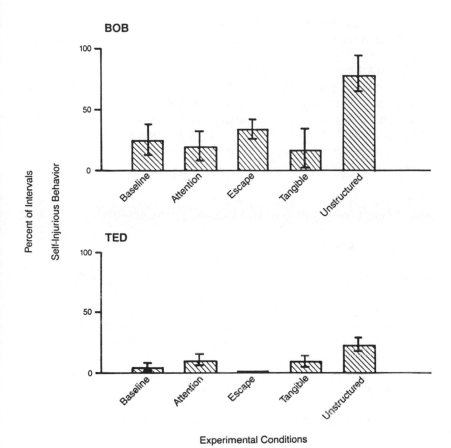

FIGURE 3-9. The percentage of self-injurious behavior in each experimental condition exhibited by the two students (Bob and Ted) rated as having "sensory-maintained" self-injury on the MAS. From "Identifying the Variables Maintaining Self-Injurious Behavior" by V. M. Durand and D. B. Crimmins, 1988, *Journal of Autism and Developmental Disorders, 18,* pp. 110–113. Copyright 1988 by Plenum Publishing Corporation. Reprinted by permission of the authors and publisher.

SUBSEQUENT RESEARCH WITH THE MAS

A number of other studies have employed the MAS to assess the variables maintaining problem behavior. For example, the MAS has been used to assess behaviors such as aggression, tantrums, and severe self-injury, with that information resulting in the design of successful interventions (e.g., Bird et al., 1989; Durand & Carr, in press; Durand & Kishi, 1987; Hall, Laitinen, & Mozzoni, 1985). The MAS was used in one study to assess the variables maintaining dangerous climbing (Swahn, 1988). In addition, we have recently used the scale to select reinforcers (Durand, Crimmins, Caulfield, & Taylor, 1989).

The MAS has also been adapted for use with individuals not having severe disabilities. For example, a modified version was recently developed to assess the environmental factors involved in pediatric headaches (Budd & Kedesdy, 1989). And, another adaptation has been used to assess the influences on children's school refusal (Kearney & Silverman, 1988). Taken together, these studies support the validity of the MAS as a tool for assessing influences on problem behavior.

Retrospective Information from Modified Environments

REVIEW OF AVAILABLE RECORDS

An additional method of assessing severe behavior problems is the review of available records. A variety of routine records are maintained by most programs, which may be of some help in assessment. Daily logs, for example, are kept in many residential programs and may serve as a source of informal information about the relationship among specific incidents and locations, staffing patterns or times of the day. Unfortunately, they rarely report information in a standardized format so that consistent themes are sometimes difficult to determine because of the different reporting styles of multiple recorders.

One source of data that captures the seriousness of a behavior is official incident reports. (e.g., Berkman & Meyer, 1988; Meyer & Evans, 1989) These documents usually follow a standard format and are submitted to a supervisor or organizational committee for review. They are useful because the occasions when they are completed are defined by organizational policies, usually in the case of injury or significant property destruction. Information presented contains a description of the incident and the circumstances surrounding it. Because their use is prescribed, they can serve as a relatively unbiased source of information. Their usefulness is, however, limited to relatively severe behaviors with serious outcomes.

Routine evaluation reports from the professional staff (e.g., psychologists, teachers, social workers, speech and language pathologists) working most closely with the individual are another potential source of information. These are, however, often limited in the degree to which they address possible functions of behavior problems. They can be helpful in describing, for example, an individual's patterns of social relationships, general communication skills, responses to frustration, and skills at occupying free time. They may also convey a sense of the *environment expectations* and a general sense of whether an individual is perceived as making progress.

Another important set of considerations that can be addressed by reviewing available records relate to *whether a behavior has recently emerged or is long-term.* A behavior problem that has only recently been observed is more likely to be viewed as reactive to a recent change in the individual's life. Although it is often acknowledged that behavior problems can be reactive to significant life events, these may not be systematically considered in planning for some individuals.

A person who has recently experienced the death of a family member may have a reactive depression that is reflected in a significant behavioral change. An intervention plan might involve a short term of supportive counseling rather than an extended behavioral plan. (e.g., Gibson, Walker, Crimmins, & Griggs, 1988).

Severe behavior problems of long standing are likely to have been addressed by numerous (and sometimes contradictory) intervention plans. Some may have been fully successful, others unsuccessful. For *successful interventions*, it is important to establish why the plan was initially successful, why it no longer is, and whether modifications of the original plan are likely to succeed. For *unsuccessful plans*, it is important to determine what effect they had on the occurrence of the behavior (i.e., did it get worse or remain the same?).

We are very interested in previous unsuccessful attempts at addressing a behavior. We have more than once encountered the response to questions about previous efforts at reducing the frequency of a behavior problem with, "I tried behavior modification and it didn't work." In avoiding philosophical discussions about behavior theory (for the sake of problem solving), we ask what happened when they "tried behavior modification." If a time-out procedure was used, for example, and a behavior became more problematic, we would begin to ask questions about the relative value of being in time-out versus being in the environment. If it was clear that time-out served as a means of avoiding demands, we would hypothesize that the behavior was escape motivated.

Existing records can also indicate *health concerns* that might contribute to the occurrence of a problem behavior. Chronic otitis media and allergy are two common conditions that may contribute to the occurrence of a problem behavior. Some medications, for some individuals, have known side-effects related to problem behavior. In other cases the compliance of an individual and his or her family with a medication regimen may affect the occurrence of a behavior.

Reviewing existing records can be helpful to some degree in assessing severe problem behaviors. *These records are likely to convey a sense of the history and context for a behavior.* Existing records are not typically directed toward the assessment of the function of a problem behavior. Thus, their utility is in identifying other considerations that may be influencing the individual.

Concurrent Information from Intact Environments

INFORMAL OBSERVATION

First efforts at assessment of a behavior often focus on informal observation and discussion of the problem with caregivers in an effort to *develop initial hypotheses about the function of a problem behavior.* The initial observation would minimally consist of some period of time in one or more environments where the behavior is likely to occur. It would also include an examination of the appropriateness of the individual's overall plan of activities and the environment. These methods may lead to a preliminary formulation of how the behavior might be maintained in the context of an interaction among the individual's capabilities, the types of interactions among that person and caregivers or peers, and qualities of the environment. This information may, in turn, lead to an initial set of recommendations that are never formalized, and, in our experience, may or may not be implemented. The question of whether this type of assessment will lead to the development of a plan for a behavior depends on a number of factors, including the skills of the caregiver in incorporating suggestions into an ongoing structure and the degree of organizational commitment to provide follow-up support during the implementation phase. Caution must be exercised regarding the potential of a plan developed in this manner.

The data-gathering process for informal assessment is subject to bias and reactivity from a number of sources. For example, caregivers may be very concerned about an individual's aggression. However, an interview conducted on the day of an injury-causing aggressive incident might lead to very different impressions than one conducted on a "good day." Knowledgeable informants can be asked why they think the behavior is occurring in an effort to obtain their hypotheses of the function of a given behavior. These intuitive hypotheses, however, are often not validated by more formal assessment procedures (Durand & Crimmins, 1988). Teachers, for example, are generally aware of the role of social attention in the acquisition and maintenance of problem behaviors. They may also report that a behavior is occurring to "get attention" when this is not supported by other observations or more extensive analysis. This may be due in part to the observation that most teachers now receive training on the role of attention, but may receive less training on the role of other consequences.

Another source of reactivity in this process is the presence of the informal observer in the environment. One cannot witness a truly random sample of behavior when the individual, peers and caregivers are all aware of the observer. With longer and/or more frequent observation periods this effect can be diminished. Informal observations may also be subject to a type of sampling error. We might witness a series of behaviors that appear to be attention seeking, yet the behaviors may not be typical of the individual. In forming recommendations, however, we are very likely to be influenced by what was seen.

Environmental observation may reveal that individuals are being asked to participate in activities that are uninteresting even to the casual observer. Or, individuals may live in understimulating environments where few attempts are made at engaging the individual in a variety of tasks. Environments may also be very chaotic. Challenging behaviors that occur under these circumstances are best responded to by providing appropriate stimulation, challenges, choices and control over the environment. Our preliminary recommendations for intervention in such cases may consist of suggestions to change the types of activities with which the person is presented or to make the environment more stimulating. Interestingly, the potential bias or reactivity in environmental observation is for it being presented at its best. Most caregivers want to present themselves as providing a responsive, structured, and stimulating environment. When that is not observed, recommendations along the lines of establishing such an environment may be well founded.

There are limits on the utility of informal observation in developing intervention recommendations for individuals. This procedure is potentially subject to bias from a number of sources that suggest caution as the best course of action. This procedure is, however, potentially useful in making a number of suggestions about the environment in which the behavior is occurring.

FORMAL OBSERVATION

Direct observation of behavior is perhaps the most common means of collecting information about maintaining variables in preparation for developing a behavior plan (see Table 3-1). These observations are typically carried out by persons in the environment with the individual who displays challenging behavior. They are, therefore, less prone to problems with reactivity noted in the section on informal observation. They are potentially limited in their usefulness by the degree of compliance with the observation procedure by the caregivers. Because observation procedures require time to carry out, they compete with other responsibilities of caregivers and are subject to sampling biases that only very salient events are recorded or that observations are reliably performed on "not busy days."

Within this general category of procedures, the direct observation of antecedents and consequences (Bijou, Peterson, & Ault, 1968) is most often used (see Figure 3-10 for example). Evans and Meyer (1985), for example, describe a formalized procedure (ABC charts) for recording each instance of a behavior (e.g., hand biting), its antecedent (e.g., teacher presented new task), and the consequence (e.g., teacher walked away). Another example of this approach is provided by Groden (1989), who describes a detailed behavioral report that requests that a target behavior, immediate and distant

ANTECEDENT	BEHAVIOR	CONSEQUENCE

FIGURE 3-10. An Antecedent–Behavior–Consequence chart.

antecedents, and different classes of consequences be specified for each occurrence of a behavior. These observation methods presume that over time a pattern will emerge that reveals the relationship between the behavior and either a specific or general class of antecedents and/or consequences. As mentioned before, these methods do require relatively good compliance in terms of accuracy and completeness of the information to provide a complete record of the behavior and its possible controlling variables.

Although ABC charts and other methods of conducting direct observation enjoy wide popularity, their reliability and validity are rarely assessed. For example, Figure 3-10 shows a typical chart used by many teachers and other caregivers to determine patterns in behavior and the environment. Space is provided for recording each instance of the problem behavior, its antecedent, and its consequence. However, Figure 3-11 illustrates how untrained and/or extremely busy individuals often complete such charts. Often no obvious antecedents are observed ("Nothing"), and poorly described consequences are recorded. Does "I ignored" mean that the teacher continued to work with the girl despite the hitting and screaming? Does it mean that the teacher walked away, or turned away? Such information is important, yet often becomes obscured in the day-to-day events. Again, information from ABC charts can be helpful, especially if used in combination with other forms of assessment.

SCATTER PLOT

An alternative direct observation procedure that is somewhat easier to complete is described by Touchette and colleagues (Touchette, MacDonald, & Langer, 1985). These authors suggest the use of a data collection procedure called a "scatter plot" that provides general information concerning the distribution of incidents of a problem behavior across the day (see Figure 3-12). The procedure is somewhat easier to complete because it requires only a categorization of the number of incidents (e.g., none, one to three, four or more) during a unit time (e.g., one half hour) rather than an absolute count and documentation of each incident. Further analysis of times of the day during which behaviors are particularly likely allows for the assessment of potential maintaining variables correlated with that time of day. For example, if the scatter plot shows that a behavior occurs during a one hour period from noon to 1 P.M., the follow-up analysis would focus on events unique to that time period—perhaps environmental conditions in the cafeteria, the opportunities for using time following lunch, and so on. Identified variables can be manipulated to determine their effect on the behavior. Touchette and his colleagues provide some initial reliability and validity data for this method (Touchette et al., 1985).

ANTECEDENT	BEHAVIOR	CONSEQUENCE
Nothing	She Screamed	I ignored
Nothing	she hit	I ignored
Nothing	she hit	I ignored
Nothing	she hit	I ignored
Nothing	she screamd	I ignored
｜（	｜（	｜｜
｜（	（（	（｜
｜（	｜（	｜｜
｜｜	she hit	｜｜
｜｜	｜（	｜｜
｜（	｜｜	｜｜
｜｜	｜｜	｜｜
｜｜	｜｜	｜｜
｜｜	｜（	｜｜

FIGURE 3-11. A completed Antecedent–Behavior–Consequence chart.

Despite the widespread use of direct observation as an assessment procedure, however, direct observation often provides little useful information about maintaining variables. One reason for the lack of information obtained from direct observation is the myriad of variables that may be involved in the maintenance of an individual's problem behavior. For example, if a teacher approaches a male student, and the student hits himself, one antecedent may be the approach of the teacher. However, other activities ongoing in the classroom (e.g., another student's yelling, the temperature of the room, the task the student has before him) or outside of the classroom (e.g., noises from children playing outside, a door closing, someone walking by a window) may have also been important antecedents to this boy's self-injury. Similarly, a range of consequences may occur beyond the one recorded during the observation. For example, if it was recorded that the consequence for this behavior was that the teacher turned and walked away from the child, then we might begin to hypothesize that escape from teacher demands is an important variable for this student. However, other consequences may be active in the maintenance of the behavior (e.g., other children in the class laughed, an assistant in the classroom gave the student a toy to calm himself, the student continued to hit himself). This is clearly a complex process and, unfortunately, *there are few guidelines available to assist individuals in selecting among the variables possibly controlling problematic behavior.*

SETTING EVENT CHECKLIST

One of the few devices specifically designed to assess *setting events* has been developed by Gardner and his associates (Gardner et al., 1986). Figure 3-13 shows the questions assessed to determine the influences of such factors as previous negative interactions, medication changes, or illness on behavior problems. Again, this checklist is unique in its attempt to assess more global influences on behavior problems. Several studies have been conducted with this device, and suggest that this information can improve the predictability of assessing behaviors such as aggression (Gardner, et al., 1986; Gardner, Karan, & Cole, 1984).

Concurrent Information from Modified Environments

ANALOGUE ASSESSMENT

A set of procedures that do offer guidelines on methods of identifying specific variables for consideration are described as analogue assessments.

Student: _____ Starting Date: _____

Day/Time	1	2	3	4	5	6	7	8	9	10	11	12	13	14	15	16	17	18	19	20	21
7:00a																					
7:30																					
8:00																					
8:30																					
9:00																					
9:30																					
10:00																					
10:30																					
11:00																					
11:30																					
12:00																					
12:30																					
1:00p																					
1:30																					
2:00																					
2:30																					

3:00																					
3:30																					
4:00																					
4:30																					
5:00																					
5:30																					
6:00																					
6:30																					
7:00																					
7:30																					
8:00																					
8:30																					
9:00																					
9:30																					
10:00																					
10:30																					

FIGURE 3-12. Scatter plot data collection sheet used for assessing time/activity patterns in challenging behavior. From "A Scatter Plot for Identifying Stimulus Control of Problem Behavior" by P. E. Touchette, R. F. MacDonald, and S. N. Langer, 1985, *Journal of Applied Behavior Analysis, 18*, p. 344. Copyright 1985 by the Society for the Experimental Analysis of Behavior, Inc. Reprinted by permission of the authors and publisher.

Client: _____ Date: _____ Completed by: _____

Check any of the following events that occurred last evening (pm) or this morning prior to work (am).

	AM	PM
Was informed of something unusually disappointing	__	__
Was refused some requested object/activity	__	__
Fought, argued, or had negative interaction(s)	__	__
Was disciplined/reprimanded (behavior or disciplinary action was atypical)	__	__
Was hurried or rushed more than usual	__	__
Sleep pattern (including duration) was unusual	__	__
Was under the care of someone new/favorite caretaker was absent	__	__
Experienced other major changes in living environment	__	__
Learned about visit/vacation with family/friends (will or will not occur)	__	__
Visitors arrived/failed to arrive	__	__
Medications were changed/missed	__	__
Has menstrual period	__	__
Appeared excessively tired/lethargic	__	__
Appeared excessively agitated	__	__
Appeared to be in bad mood	__	__
Appeared/complained of being ill	__	__
Other (_____)	__	__

FIGURE 3-13. Setting Event Checklist. From "Reducing Aggression in Individuals with Developmental Disabilities: An Expanded Stimulus Control, Assessment, and Intervention Model" by W. I. Gardner, C. L. Cole, D. P. Davidson, and O. C. Karan, 1986, *Education and Training of the Mentally Retarded, 21,* p. 7. Copyright 1986 by Education and Training of the Mentally Retarded. Reprinted by permission of the authors and publisher.

These assessments involve the manipulation of various antecedents and consequences that are presumed to be important and observing their effect on an individual's problem behavior. Carr and Durand (1985a) and Iwata et al. (1982) provide examples of this type of work. Iwata and colleagues, for example, devised a series of analogue conditions to determine the role of social attention, sensory consequences, and task demands on the self-injury of nine individuals. They found considerable variability both within and between the individuals observed in these conditions, suggesting that self-injurious behavior may be a function of different consequences. Similarly, Carr and Durand (1985a) observed that low levels of adult attention and high task demands were discriminative for problem behavior in four children with developmental disabilities. Providing the children with alternative verbal responses based on the assessment findings (Functional Communication Training) resulted in significant reductions in aggression, self-injury, and tantrums. Knowledge of the role of these variables was predictive of intervention outcome.

We recently designed four analogue conditions to assess for the separate influence of social attention, tangible consequences, escape/avoidance, and sensory consequences as maintaining variables for the self-injurious behavior of eight children with developmental disabilities (Durand & Crimmins, 1988). Each of the four analogue conditions was contrasted with the behavior of the children in a baseline period that attempted to create a highly reinforcing environment with presumed minimal rate of problem behaviors. The characteristics of the baseline session were that there was a relatively easy task, with contingent access to high rates of social attention and tangible rewards. The four analogue conditions varied from the baseline by the removal/reduction of one key element. For example, in assessing for the influence of social attention, teacher attention was available at one third the rate of the baseline.

The other three analogue conditions involved increasing task difficulty to assess for escape/avoidance, reducing the rate of tangible rewards to assess for their influence, and reducing the structure of the session to assess for sensory behaviors. Each of the five analogue assessment conditions was presented three times. This procedure can be seen as a relatively time-consuming and complex undertaking.

Although these procedures are complex, one can adapt them for use in real-life environments. We encourage caregivers to identify potential variables and conduct brief instructional interactions that systematically provide and remove the variable in question. In this way a less formal assessment of maintaining variables can be attempted.

Another procedure derived from analogue assessment techniques is to ask caregivers to set up some set of conditions that minimize the occurrence of the behavior problem. We generally approach this by asking teachers or caregivers what they would have to do to have a period (the length of the period is relative to the base rate of the behavior; it might vary from 5 minutes to a day) in which the behavior would be very *unlikely to occur.* Responses often fall into the categories mentioned in our discussion of maintaining variables: "If I just let him eat, he'd be fine," "If I paid attention only to her, she'd be great," "If I just left him to do his own thing, there would be no problem," "If I never asked her to do anything, she would be okay." We then ask the caregivers to attempt to set up these conditions. In this way caregivers can have the experience of demonstrating stimulus control over the behavior. This has two useful outcomes. First, caregivers who feel that a behavior problem is totally beyond control or remediation are faced with contradictory information. Second, *this procedure identifies a situation that might be an appropriate starting place for an intervention.*

Although constructing analogue situations in order to observe changes in problem behavior may be a valid way of assessing maintaining variables, this approach has several drawbacks. First, several highly trained staff members are usually employed in these studies, necessitating extra personnel. Second, these assessments can take several days, weeks, or even months, and this delay may be unacceptable in certain crisis situations. Third, there are times when the problem behavior is so dangerous that no instances of the behavior can be tolerated. Derivations from these procedures can be helpful but often face the same obstacles as direct observation procedures mentioned previously: Guidelines on identifying relevant variables for assessment are not widely available.

Summary

As mentioned on numerous occasions previously, there is no *one* correct way to assess the variables maintaining problem behavior. There will always be tradeoffs between the amount of effort employed in conducting these assessments, and the quality of information received. Less formal methods can be advantageous in generating hypotheses. However, these hypotheses should always be confirmed by information collected from more formal assessment methods. Again, our rule of thumb has been to use two or more formal assessment methods, preferably ones with some data available on reliability and validity. We usually use the MAS and one other method (e.g., analogues, ABC charts) to lend credibility to or refute our initial impressions. Our next step becomes selecting the reinforcer(s) to be used during our skills training efforts. The next section covers methods to select these reinforcers.

Reinforcer Assessment

In our search for optimal habilitation procedures for persons with severe developmental disabilities, the issue of motivation is ever present. Concern for providing the most effective reinforcers spans diagnostic category (e.g., Infantile Autism: Koegel & Mentis, 1985; Mental Retardation: Zigler & Balla, 1977) and target of training (e.g., language: Goetz, Schuler, & Sailor, 1983; academic performance: Konarski, Crowell, Johnson, & Whitman,

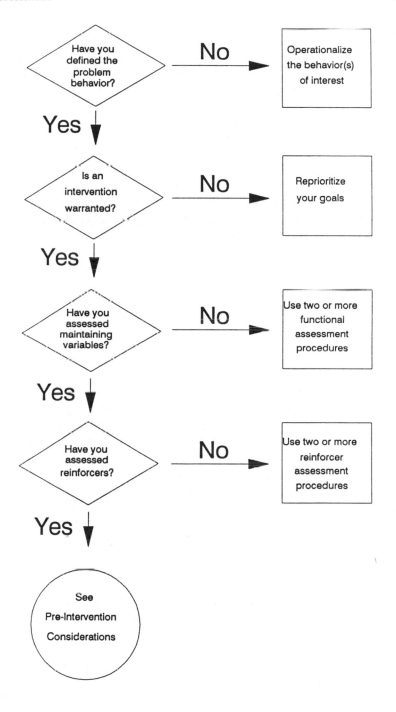

1982). Given the behavioral/educational model that currently pervades the intervention of persons with severe developmental disabilities (Lovaas, Koegel, Simmons, & Long, 1973; Schopler, Brehm, Kinsbourne, & Reichler, 1971), understanding the nature of the reinforcers used with these individuals seems particularly important.

In this section, we discuss the vital job of selecting reinforcers. Given the educational nature of nonaversive interventions, it is critical that powerful reinforcers be identified. Effective reinforcers are integral to the process of teaching new skills. And, it is doubtful that significant behavior change can occur without identifying and using one or more potent reinforcers. Fortunately, there has been a recent increase in research on reinforcer selection and use. Following some discussion of reinforcer terminology, we review the recent efforts pertaining to assessing reinforcers for individuals with developmental disabilities.

Terminology

A physics teacher once taught this writer a lesson in terminology that has had a lasting influence. A group of students were discussing the difference between joules and ergs (units of work or energy—a joule equals 10,000,000 ergs) during class time; some fellow students were being chastised if they confused the terms. Our teacher interrupted angrily, saying that we were wasting our time. He pointed out that it really didn't matter if we labeled our results "joules," "ergs," or even "potatoes" as long as we defined what it was we meant (e.g., foot-pounds). After that exchange, our use of creative terms increased (one favorite was "strain"), but so did our accuracy in defining our terms ("force times distance").

In the current context, there are a number of terms being used as descriptors for reinforcers. Words such as "natural," "functional," "preferred," and "arbitrary" have been used in various contexts in the literature. Unfortunately, the terms are sometimes used without definition, or are used differently by different authors. Therefore, this discussion of reinforcer assessment will include an examination of the terms used to describe reinforcers. *We have decided to label stimuli to be used as reinforcers on the basis of how they are chosen.* In other words, instead of attempting to define these stimuli based on how we believe they may be related to the student and his or her behavior, we have labeled them based on the reasoning for their selection. This may seem to be a minor distinction, however, it should soon become clear that this approach avoids assumptions that may lead to later problems. Therefore, although there are any number of ways to categorize reinforcers (see, for example, Ferster, 1965; Konarski, Johnson, Crowell, & Whitman, 1981; Premack, 1959,

1965, 1971; Rusch, Rose, & Greenwood, 1988), we have used the guide illustrated in Table 3-2 to assist us in selecting reinforcers for the persons with whom we work.

Logical Stimuli

Some stimuli used as reinforcers are directly related to the target response or are usually observed as consequences for these behaviors in the prevailing environment. Caregivers and educators select them because they follow logically from the type of response being taught. These stimuli, if effective, are preferred for use when teaching skills. For example, putting on a coat is usually followed by increased warmth. And, if it is cold outside, putting on a coat might be reinforcing. Making a request such as "I want soda" is typically followed by access to soda. Learning to turn a doorknob results in access to new rooms. The stimuli in these response–stimulus chains are examples of what we might refer to as a logical stimuli. If, in the above examples, putting on coats, making the request, and turning door knobs each increase in probability, then we could say they were reinforced. We call them *logical stimuli* because they are consequences that typically follow the target responses. They are logically related to the response being taught.

What we are labeling as logical stimuli have sometimes been referred to as *natural* (e.g., Donnellan & Mirenda, 1983; Ferster, Culbertson, & Boren, 1975; Koegel & Johnson, 1989; Neel & Billingsley, 1989), *functional* (e.g., Williams, Koegel, & Egel, 1981), or *direct* (Koegel & Williams, 1980). The difference in labeling is related to the different categorization system being used here. The use of terms such as natural, functional, or direct has typically been based on the presumed relationship between the stimuli and the environment ("natural") or the response ("functional," "direct"). As was mentioned before, we have decided to label reinforcers based on how they are chosen, because this avoids any presumption about the nature of these relationships.

TABLE 3-2. Type of stimuli used as reinforcers

Logical Stimuli	Stimuli that are selected based on their relationship to the targeted response or the prevailing environment
Preferred Stimuli	Stimuli that are selected based on the presumed preference of the student
Functional Stimuli	Stimuli selected because they presumably are functionally related to the student's behavior.

SELECTING LOGICAL STIMULI

There are currently no formal assessment procedures for selecting logical stimuli to be used as reinforcers. However, the following are guidelines to provide readers with suggestions for ways of selecting these stimuli.

   1. *Select a stimulus that typically follows the targeted behavior in the setting in which you want it to occur.* For example, if you want to teach a verbal request (such as "May I have something to drink?"), the stimulus you would choose as a consequence should be the one provided by the person who would most likely be asked the request (e.g., mother who provides a glass of milk).
   2. *Select a stimulus that can be inserted in the teaching situation such that it will immediately follow the targeted behavior.* An illustration of this principle would be to teach opening a jar by placing in it a favorite food or toy that the student can have access to once the jar is opened (e.g., Koegel & Williams, 1980).
   3. *Select a stimulus that has information value to the student.* One aspect of relevance involves the *information value* of the reinforcer. In other words, does the reinforcer in some way assist in identifying the correct response? For example, praise that has informational value might involve phrases such as, "Great! Thank you for picking up your clothes," where the desired behavior was cleaning up the room. Several studies have demonstrated the value of using stimuli with informational value over stimuli that do not have informational value (e.g., Litt & Schreibman, 1982; Saunders & Sailor, 1979).

   It has sometimes been said that one should select a stimulus as a reinforcer because it is the "natural consequence" in the environment. For example, as noted above, if you want to teach opening a jar to improve motor skills, then it makes sense to have a favorite food in the jar to be consumed by the student after it is opened. However, finding a favorite food in a jar being opened isn't always the natural consequence. The other day, this writer asked his son to open a jar of pickles, which he did. Why did he open the jar of pickles? Does he like pickles? No. He probably opened it because he was asked, and because in the past the consequence for doing this was social attention (i.e., a smile from his father and the phrase, "Thanks for your help, pal!").
   In the previous example, the natural consequence was approval. However, as those of us who work with persons with severe disabilities know all too well, approval alone isn't always an effective reinforcer for these individuals. *There are many times when the consequence that they are likely to receive in the prevailing environment will not be sufficient to teach or*

maintain a behavior. For example, many social-communicative behaviors (e.g., saying the phrase, "Hi, how are you?") are followed by extended social interaction (e.g., another person saying, "I'm fine, how are you doing?"). Yet, there are individuals who do not prefer social interactions, and for some, these can even serve as a punisher (e.g., Durand et al., 1989; Herbert et al., 1973). In this case, the natural consequence to communication will not serve to encourage future interactions. In fact, the natural consequence may actively *discourage* future instances of the desired behavior. At this point, many educators and others often turn to stimuli that the student appears to prefer to be used as reinforcers.

Preferred Stimuli

As mentioned above, if possible, logical stimuli are favored as task reinforcers. Yet, there are times when these stimuli are not effective reinforcers. When this situation occurs, those involved look to the student for other stimuli that might serve as reinforcers. Based on a variety observations, caregivers attempt to determine those stimuli preferred by the student. *It is assumed, then, that if the student prefers a particular stimulus (e.g., a favorite toy), that stimulus should serve as a reinforcer.*

SELECTING PREFERRED STIMULI

If the student is successful in using some form of communication, then one means of obtaining this information is to ask the student. However, there are many students who cannot or do not express preferences. Fortunately, several methods of selecting stimuli to be used as reinforcers based on student preference exist, and there has been some recent research on the use of some of these procedures. Table 3-3 lists and critiques procedures used to select preferred stimuli, as well as logical stimuli (discussed previously) and functional stimuli (to be discussed next).

INTUITIVE SELECTION

Perhaps the most common method of selecting reinforcers is through *intuitive selection procedures* (e.g., Mullins & Rincover, 1985). As was true for the assessment of the function of behavior problems previously discussed, caregivers typically determine what a student likes or prefers by relying on informal observations. Sometimes this is accomplished by selecting stimuli that have been effective with other, similar students. Others determine

Table 3-3. Reinforcer selection methods

Procedure	Example	Advantages	Disadvantages
Logical stimuli	(See guidelines in Reinforcer Assessment section of Chapter 3, this volume)	Most likely to be available in the prevailing environment Often has information value to the student May facilitate generalization and maintenance	May not always follow response in the environment Such stimuli may not serve as reinforcers Selection methods have no demonstrated reliability and validity
Preferred stimuli			
Intuitive selection	Mullins & Rincover, 1985	Selection method is easy to use Face validity	Selection methods have no demonstrated reliability or validity Such stimuli may not always serve as reinforcers
Surveys	Atkinson et al., 1984	Surveys are easy to administer More formalized method of selecting from a variety of stimuli Some methods have reliability data	Such stimuli may not always serve as reinforcers Little validity data available
Pretesting	Green et al., 1988; Pace et al., 1983	Detects preference differences over time Reliability and validity data available for some methods	Selected stimuli may not serve as reinforcers Some students do not demonstrate preferences
Functional stimuli			
High probability behavior	Osborne, 1969	Directly related student behavior Useful when student does not express preferences	No demonstrated reliability Little validity data available Not practical with severe behavior problems
Stimuli associated with high probability behavior	Durand et al., 1989	Directly related to student behavior Useful when student does not express preferences Reliability and validity available	Stimuli may not be available in prevailing environment

preference by observing reactions such as smiles or proximity to certain stimuli. These methods of determining preference suffer from inadequate reliability and validity, and because of this, more formal selection methods have been developed.

SURVEYS

One additional method of determining reinforcer preference is to ask caregivers to list those consequences that seem to serve as reinforcers for particular students by means of a *survey*. In one study (Atkinson et al., 1984), staff members at a clinic were asked to complete the Autism Reinforcer Checklist for children with autism. These responses were compared with the responses by the children's mothers and were found to be highly correlated. Thus, staff and parents agreed on what would be reinforcing for students. A problem with this analysis is that it assumes that staff and/or parents can accurately determine the reinforcer preferences of students. Recent research suggests that this may not always be true (Green et al., 1988). In addition, any validation of a reinforcer selection procedure should involve a demonstration of the use of selected consequences on student behavior. To date, no surveys have been validated by this method.

PRETESTING

Recently, some workers have gone to the systematic *pretesting of stimuli* to determine their reinforcing properties (e.g., Datillo, 1986; Dyer, 1987; Green et al., 1988; Mason, McGee, Farmer–Dougan, & Risley, 1989; Pace, Ivancic, Edwards, Iwata, & Page, 1985; Reid & Hurlbut, 1977; Wacker, Berg, Wiggins, Muldoon, & Cavanaugh, 1985; Wuerch & Voeltz, 1982). For example, Dyer (1987) assessed stimulus preference each day prior to teaching sessions. Objects were introduced to students one by one, and were rated by observers using specific criteria. These criteria are outlined in the Preference Assessment shown in Figure 3-14.

Dyer found that for most students, preferred stimuli served as reinforcers. However, for some students in this study and in others (e.g., Pace et al., 1985), stimuli that were preferred *did not* serve as reinforcers. And, Green and her colleagues have found that *some students do not show preferences with such systematic assessments* (Green et al., 1988). Although this appears counterintuitive, some students do not express preferences, and for those who do, sometimes these stimuli do not serve

Student Name: _____
Teacher/Date: _____

Preference Assessment

Introduce the object to the student and demonstrate how it can be manipulated, then, rate the object according to the following criteria of student behaviors:

1. Student manipulates object for more that 15 seconds without prompting from therapist.

2. Student resists when therapists attempts to take object from student.

3. When object is taken away from student and placed about one foot away, student reaches for object within 3 seconds (Actual physical movement or shifts gaze between object and therapist).

4. Student exhibits positive affect while manipulating the object (smiles, laughs, or looks absorbed).

If the student demonstrates three or more of the above behaviors, it is a preferred object.

If a student shows an interest in a non-assessed item during the day, assess it. If a student becomes bored with an assessed preferred activity, discontinue using that item and assess a new item. Behaviors associated with boredom are:

a) looking away from activity
b) changing subject or asking for something else
c) engaging in self-stimulation
d) stopping activity

Item or Activity	Manipulates object 15 seconds	Resists	Reaches w/in 3 seconds	Positive Affect

FIGURE 3-14. The format used by Dyer (1987) to assess stimulus preference. From "The Competition of Autistic Stereotyped Behavior with Usual and Specially Assessed Reinforcers" by K. Dyer, 1987, *Research in Developmental Disabilities, 8,* pp. 607–626. Copyright 1987 by Kathleen Dyer, PhD. Reprinted by permission.

as reinforcers. Recently, researchers have explored ways to teach choice making, and readers are directed to some of this work for further assistance in this area (e.g., Guess & Siegel–Causey, 1985; Peck, 1985; Wuerch & Voeltz, 1982). However, when the stimuli students do choose do not serve as powerful reinforcers, then an additional approach is to select functional stimuli.

Functional Stimuli

When both logical and preferred stimuli prove less than optimal as reinforcers, an additional method of choosing stimuli can be used. Selecting stimuli based on their observed relationship to the student's behavior will be referred to as picking *functional stimuli*. The basic premise of this approach is: If you want to find out what people like, look at what they do. If someone asked what would be a good reinforcer for me in my office, probably the last thing I would think of to choose would be to spend time writing in front of my computer. Yet, if you observed me over long periods of time in the office, undoubtedly the vast majority of my time would be spent doing just that. So, although I might not verbalize writing as a reinforcer, it is reasonable to assume that giving me access to the computer for this purpose would reinforce any behavior it followed. Two ways of selecting functional stimuli are discussed below.

SELECTING FUNCTIONAL STIMULI

Perhaps the most conventional method of selecting these stimuli is commonly referred to as the "Premack Principle." This principle states that a high probability response can be used to reinforce a low probability response (Premack, 1959). For example, if you want to reinforce working at a table (low probability response), you could follow periods of work with activities available during free time (high probability response) (Osborne, 1969). The assessment process therefore involves assessing the probability of the target behavior (i.e., the low probability response you want to increase), and finding another response that has a high probability of occurring. This latter response then becomes the reinforcer (Allen & Iwata, 1980; Homme, de Baca, Devine, Steinhorst, & Rickert, 1963; Koegel, Dyer, & Bell, 1987; Mitchell & Stoffelmayr, 1973).

One interesting outcome of this type of work has been the attempt by some workers to use the high probability problem behaviors themselves as reinforcers. For example, Wolery, Kirk, and Gast (1985) found that by cuing students to engage in their noninjurious stereotyped behaviors (e.g., licking

fingers, playing with saliva) following correct responses, their task performance increased. They also found that these stereotyped behaviors did not
increase. These findings have now been replicated by a number of researchers (e.g., Charlop, Kurtz, & Casey, 1989; Hung, 1978; Wolery, 1978).
There are several problems to recommending this approach to reinforcer
selection. First, although most of the studies in this area report no increase
in the behaviors used as reinforcers, there is also no reported *decrease*
(occasional exceptions are noted by Charlop et al., 1989). This will be a
problem if the goal is the eventual reduction of these behaviors. A second
problem involves the use of high probability challenging behavior when
these behaviors can potentially cause injury or will result in stigmatization
in the community. *It is obvious that behaviors such as severe aggression or
self-injury could not be encouraged for use as reinforcers.*

However, a second approach to selecting functional stimuli makes use
of challenging behavior in a way that is not harmful to the student or others.
We have recently used *the stimuli associated with high probability responses*
as reinforcers (Durand et al., 1989). In other words, we select high probability responses (in this case, behaviors such as aggression, self-injury, and
tantrums) and assess the variables maintaining them. So, for example, if we
found that a student's hand biting was maintained by adult attention, then
we could assume that adult attention (e.g., social praise) would serve as a
reinforcer for this student. Similarly, if a second student's hand biting was
maintained by escape from demands, then removing task demands contingent upon some desired behavior could serve as a reinforcer. Therefore,
instead of using the problem behavior itself as a reinforcer, we determine
why the student engaged in that behavior, and use that information to select
reinforcers.

Assessing for reinforcers in this way is accomplished in the same way
we assess the function of behavior problems (see above in section on
"Assessing Influences on Problem Behavior"). We usually select one or two
of the most frequent behavior problems in the person's repertoire to be
assessed, and typically use the MAS and one other form of assessment to
determine possible controlling variables. For example, Figure 3-15 shows
responses on the MAS for Bill. The results indicated that he was hitting
objects frequently, primarily to escape demands. Based on this information,
we recommended that escape in the form of ending work for a short period
of time be used as a reinforcer for him.

The use of escape as a reinforcer was implemented in the following
manner. If he completed some portion of a task correctly, then the teacher
was instructed to give him feedback (e.g., "That's really nice work") and
then remove the task for a period of time (e.g., 1–2 minutes). It was observed
that when this type of stimulus (i.e., removing work briefly) was made
contingent upon correct responses, not only did he improve his work perfor-

mance, but he also appeared happier, and engaged in fewer behavior problems during the sessions. Similar results have been observed in a number of other students (Durand et al., 1989). Thus, when stimuli are used as task consequences that are selected based on the variables maintaining their behavior problems, improvements in task performance, affect, and problem behavior are often noted.

Summary of Reinforcer Assessment

As we found in the review of methods of assessing maintaining variables, there are a variety of procedures for selecting stimuli to be used as reinforcers. And, as noted in that section, there is no one correct way to select these stimuli. Because of issues related to generalization and maintenance, it is preferred that stimuli be used that will be available in the prevailing environment. However, if these stimuli do not currently maintain performance, then the various other approaches to selecting stimuli should be used. Plans need to be made from the start of training to pair the reinforcers being used with the consequences available in the prevailing or future environment. Obviously, for the student to *use* their new skills, they will need to receive reinforcement in the settings were you want them to be exhibited.

Summary

A great deal of information is presented in this chapter on assessment. We have tried to present an overview for the different questions that should be asked, and have discussed methods for answering some of these questions. In order to make this process a little easier, flow charts are provided to summarize of the type of information you should collect about behavior problems, and recommended strategies. Once this assessment process has been followed, it is time to turn attention to a variety of preintervention considerations that will affect the ultimate intervention program. The next section discusses the final preparations needed prior to implementing functional communication training.

Name **Bill** Rater **Mark** Date **7/16/88**

Behavior Description **Hitting objects (e.g., tops of tables) with his hand.**

Setting Description **One-to-one instructional settings in school**

Instructions: The **Motivation Assessment Scale** is a questionnaire designed to identify those situations in which an individual is likely to behave in certain ways. From this information, more informed decisions can be made concerning the selection of appropriate reinforcers and treatments. To complete the **Motivation Assessment Scale**, select one behavior that is of particular interest. It is important that you identify the behavior *very specifically*. *Aggressive*, for example, is not as good a description as *hits his sister*. Once you have specified the behavior to be rated, read each question carefully and circle the *one* number that best describes your observations of this behavior.

QUESTIONS

ANSWERS

	Never	Almost Never	Seldom	Half the Time	Usually	Almost Always	Always

1. Would the behavior occur continuously, over and over, if this person was left alone for long periods of time? (For example, several hours.)

Never	Almost Never	Seldom	Half the Time	Usually	Almost Always	Always
(0)	1	2	3	4	5	6

2. Does the behavior occur following a request to perform a difficult task?

Never	Almost Never	Seldom	Half the Time	Usually	Almost Always	Always
0	1	2	3	4	(5)	6

3. Does the behavior seem to occur in response to your talking to other persons in the room?

Never	Almost Never	Seldom	Half the Time	Usually	Almost Always	Always
0	(1)	2	3	4	5	6

4. Does the behavior ever occur to get a toy, food, or activity that this person has been told that he or she can't have?

Never	Almost Never	Seldom	Half the Time	Usually	Almost Always	Always
0	1	2	(3)	4	5	6

#	Question	Never 0	Almost Never 1	Seldom 2	Half the Time 3	Usually 4	Almost Always 5	Always 6
5.	Would the behavior occur repeatedly, in the same way, for very long periods of time, if no one was around? (For example, rocking back and forth for over an hour.)	**(0)**	1	2	3	4	5	6
6.	Does the behavior occur when any request is made of this person?	0	1	2	3	**(4)**	5	6
7.	Does the behavior occur whenever you stop attending to this person?	0	**(1)**	2	3	4	5	6
8.	Does the behavior occur when you take away a favorite toy, food, or activity?	0	1	2	3	**(4)**	5	6
9.	Does it appear to you that this person enjoys performing the behavior? (It feels, tastes, looks, smells, and/or sounds pleasing.)	0	**(1)**	2	3	4	5	6
10.	Does this person seem to do the behavior to upset or annoy you when you are trying to get him or her to do what you ask?	0	1	2	3	4	5	6
11.	Does this person seem to do the behavior to upset or annoy you when you are not paying attention to him or her? (For example, if you are sitting in a separate room, interacting with another person.)	0	1	**(2)**	3	4	5	6
12.	Does the behavior stop occurring shortly after you give this person the toy, food or activity he or she has requested?	0	1	2	3	**(4)**	5	6
13.	When the behavior is occurring, does this person seem calm and unaware of anything else going on around him or her?	**(0)**	1	2	3	4	5	6

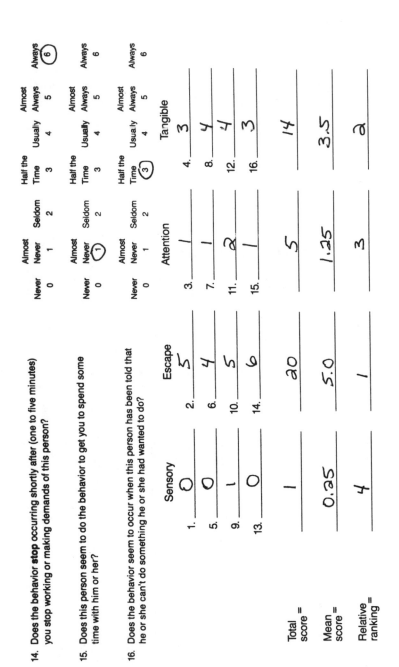

14. Does the behavior **stop** occurring shortly after (one to five minutes) you stop working or making demands of this person?

15. Does this person seem to do the behavior to get you to spend some time with him or her?

16. Does the behavior seem to occur when this person has been told that he or she can't do something he or she had wanted to do?

	Never 0	Almost Never 1	Seldom 2	Half the Time 3	Usually 4	Almost Always 5	Always 6
14.							(6)
15.		(1)					6
16.				(3)			6

Sensory		Escape		Attention		Tangible	
1.	0	2.	5	3.	1	4.	3
5.	0	6.	4	7.	1	8.	4
9.	1	10.	5	11.	2	12.	4
13.	0	14.	6	15.	1	16.	3
Total score =	1		20		5		14
Mean score =	0.25		5.0		1.25		3.5
Relative ranking =	4		1		3		2

FIGURE 3-15. A completed Motivation Assessment Scale for Bill's object hitting in one-to-one instructional settings. Reprinted by permission of V. Mark Durand, State University of New York at Albany.

4

Preintervention Considerations

The premise is simple. Teach individuals to produce a form of communication that will get them what they want in a particular situation. Because a reinforcer has already been identified (i.e., based on the reinforcer assessment procedures described in Chapter 3), successful communication training should be easy. It is not.

Obstacles to Communication Training

There are a number of reasons why the act of teaching communication to persons with severe challenging behavior is difficult. The most obvious obstacle to successful teaching is the challenging behavior itself. It is very frustrating to try to teach someone who is hitting you, is hitting oneself, or is generally disruptive in the teaching situation. In fact, this is often the rationale for using extremely restrictive procedures. It is usually assumed that no teaching can go on while the person continues to engage in disruptive behavior. Therefore, a "temporary" program is recommended, using some form of aversive consequence to reduce the frequency of the problem behavior. The reasoning continues that once the rate of problem behavior is reduced, then teaching can be carried out.

In the abstract, this rationale seems logical. Unfortunately, too often and for too many people, this scenario is played out differently. Initially, getting those involved to agree on and design a plan can take several weeks. Then, acquiring the approvals necessary to begin a plan that uses an extremely restrictive procedure can take several months. It is frequently the case that the time between program development and implementation for restrictive interventions is considerable (Matson & Kazdin, 1981). And, once caregivers have been trained and the intervention has been attempted, often there is no quick reduction in the problem behavior. What follows, then, is a series of meetings, discussions, and modifications to the intervention that can also take several months. It is not uncommon that after more than 6 months, there still is no significant reduction in the behavior problem, and no teaching of alternative behaviors.

On the other hand, there are instances when the process is much quicker. Within a relatively short period of time, the frequency of the behavior problem is substantially reduced. Unfortunately, once the crisis is over, too often so is the degree of concern for this person's continued progress. The financial and personal resources previously made available when the person was in danger or was placing others at risk are no longer forthcoming. Rarely are outside resources brought in (either before or after) to assist in designing programs to teach alternative behaviors. It is frequently the case that once the behavior problem is reduced, "phase two" (teaching alternative skills) is often ignored or carried out in a perfunctory manner.

These scenarios all presuppose that communication training (or teaching other alternative skills) can not be carried out with a person who is engaging in severe behavior problems. As the reader will see throughout the remainder of the book, *our efforts at teaching communication strategies to persons exhibiting challenging behavior have all been conducted prior to reductions in these behavior problems.* We have not waited until these behaviors were reduced or eliminated, but rather adapted our teaching efforts to continue despite the behavior of the people with whom we worked. Often, we have set up the teaching situation so that behavior problems are minimized. However, this has not always been possible, and on rare occasions, we have even taught communication strategies to persons while they were in mechanical restraints. *Challenging behavior should not be viewed as a major barrier to teaching communication.*

The previous scenarios also point out a level of analysis that has not yet been carried out systematically—*the ecology of an intervention plan.* In addition to studying the ecology of behavior problems, we also need to study the effects of using a particular intervention on how the person is subsequently treated by others. As just described, it is often the case that by quickly ending a crisis with a restraint or some contingent aversive stimulus, the level of concern for the person is reduced, as are efforts to teach alternative behaviors. It may be that acute crises can facilitate positive efforts on the part of concerned persons.

A second obstacle to teaching communication lies in the abilities of those who daily work with persons with severe handicaps. Rarely are these people provided with extensive training in how to teach communication skills. This is in contrast to efforts at teaching caregivers to implement restrictive procedures. Great care is taken to provide these people with the necessary skills to carry out properly procedures such as overcorrection, time-out, and so on (Carr & Lovaas, 1983; Foxx, Plaska, & Bittle, 1986). Yet, it is common that relatively few training resources are available to teach these same people how to fade a prompt properly, or set up the environment to encourage communicative interactions (Durand, 1987). Extraordinary effort is required to intervene successfully with severe behavior problems. This is true whether it involves training and safeguards in the use of restrictive procedures, or training and monitoring of programs involving teaching alternative skills.

Increasingly, there are staff, teachers, parents, and other involved persons who attempt to intervene in the face of severe behavior problems, and who possess excellent teaching skills. However, it bears repeating that despite the best efforts of many of these individuals, successful intervention can require extraordinary effort. Although this book attempts to provide guidelines throughout its pages, there are many decisions that must be made that have no "cookbook" answer. At times, the only choice is to be willing to keep trying creative alternatives. If faced with efforts that are not successful, readers are encouraged to consult with others both within their own existing system, and with persons from outside of their system for a fresh perspective on the problem.

A final concern expressed by some who work with persons with severe and profound handicaps is that of the necessity of teaching cognitive prerequisite skills prior to communication training. It has sometimes been argued that teaching communication skills to persons who do not have these prerequisites would be a futile effort. In our work, *we have not waited to teach these prerequisites, but instead prompted and reinforced successive approximations of these communicative responses.* We have successfully taught these skills to persons with some of the most severe handicaps, and this in turn has resulted in decreased problem behavior (Durand & Kishi, 1987). It could be argued that functional communication training involves the concurrent teaching of cognitive skills and symbolic representational skills (Schiefelbusch, 1980), because it provides experiences with communicative interactions and symbolic representations in a naturalistic context. Our data suggest that teaching such prerequisites separately may not be necessary in order to achieve rudimentary communicative competence (Durand & Kishi, 1987).

What and Where to Teach

Before beginning to teach alternate communicative responses, a number of issues must be addressed. First, once the decision has been made to begin

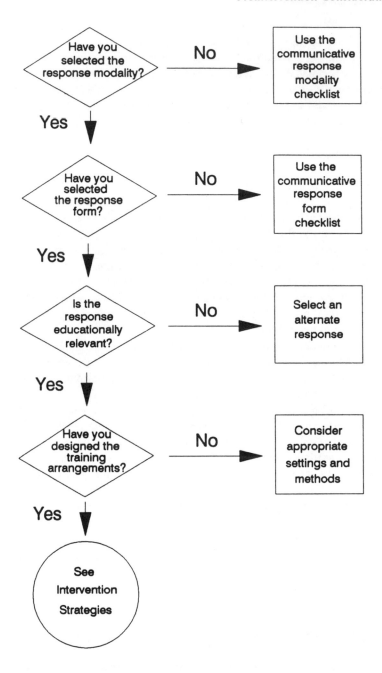

FIGURE 4-1. Preintervention considerations.

teaching communication, the next step is to determine which response to teach. Should you attempt to teach a verbal response, a manual sign, or have the student point to a picture or symbol? Also, with a student displaying escape-maintained problem behavior, should you teach him or her to request a break from work, help on a task, or for some time working alone? If the behavior of another student involves attention-getting responses, should you teach a request for a hug, a request to join a group, or a response that will get him or her in proximity to a favorite peer?

In addition to the type of response to be taught, decisions are required as to the setting or settings in which training should be carried out. Should you begin training in one setting and then expand the range of settings? Should they be conducted in the same way in every setting?

In the following section, we will address preintervention issues in detail. Our experience suggests that there is considerable variability in the way people view these training options. We will present our decision-making process, and the rationales for each decision.

Selecting a Communicative Response

Once it has been determined that a communication intervention is warranted and the proper assessments have been carried out (see Chapter 3), the next step involves selecting the response to be used for the communicative behavior and the modality in which it will be taught and used (see Figure 4-1). In what follows, we discuss guidelines for selecting the particular response to teach.

RESPONSE MODALITY

Much has been written about teaching communication in general and, specifically, selecting the modality to use for teaching. Readers interested in this issue are encouraged to refer to other sources for a more comprehensive treatment of communication training (e.g., Guess, 1980; Harris, 1975; Hart, 1981; Kent, 1974; Schiefelbusch, 1978; Yoder & Calculator, 1981) as well as selecting training modalities (e.g., see Halle, 1988; Reichle & Karlan 1985; Reichle & Yoder, 1979; Sailor et al., 1980). In general, decisions are required as to the *input* mode for teaching (i.e., how information should be provided to the student), as well as the *output* mode (i.e., how you want the student to communicate). Teaching can be accomplished by a variety of means, including through visual (e.g., signs, gestures), auditory (e.g., verbally), or tactile (e.g., physical prompts) modalities. Such decisions should

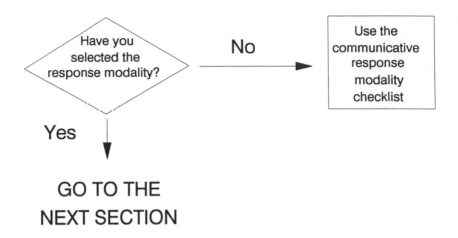

be made on the basis of the ability of the student to perceive different sensory stimuli (Sailor et al., 1980).

Similarly, the type of response to encourage from the student also needs to be determined. If the student already has some facility in one mode of communication (e.g., signing), then that mode should be considered for functional communication training. Usually, if a student has been unsuccessful in learning to communicate effectively after extensive verbal language training, then the communication modality to be used should either be signing or symbolic. If the student has also been unsuccessful with sign language training (e.g., has not learned to sign or uses "sloppy" and incomprehensible signs) we recommend symbolic communication training, at least initially. Symbolic communication training can involve the use of picture books, tokens with messages written on them, or other assistive devices (e.g., Wolf communication board, IntroTalker). This form of communication training has the advantage of being relatively easy to teach, and is universally recognizable.

The checklist presented here (in Figure 4-2) illustrates the decision-making process followed when selecting a response modality. For example, the checklist completed on Lee indicates that she has no formal communication system that is used regularly. However, she occasionally communicates her desires through gestures. These results suggest that initial functional communication training might be started using gestures. None of these is a "hard and fast" rule. As with any other clinical/educational decision, the student's particular needs and wants as well as a considerations of the prevailing environment should be evaluated. For cxample, whenever possible, the student should be given a choice of communication modes and be

Communicative Response Modality Checklist

Student's Name: _____L e e_____   Date:_ 7 / 2 2 / 89

Respondent's Name:___G l e n_____

1. Does the student use one of the following methods of communication on a regular basis? (if more than one is used, circle the preferred method)

    VERBAL   SIGN/GESTURAL   SYMBOLIC   (NO)

    If one of the above methods is circled, this may be the modality used for the communicative response. If NO is circled, go to question #2.

2. Does the student use one or more verbal responses to communicate on an occasional basis (e.g., "cookie," "no")?

                    YES   (NO)

    If YES, then the communicative response might be verbal. If NO, go to question #3.

3. Does the student use one or more signs or understandable gestures to communicate on an occasional basis?

                    (YES)   NO

    If YES, then the communicative response might be signed/gestural. If NO, go to question #4.

4. Does the student use one or more symbolic forms of communication to communicate on an occasional basis (e.g., points to pictures in a picture book)?

                    YES   NO

    If YES, then the communicative response may be symbolic. If NO, go to question #5.

5. Is one method of communication being emphasized in speech/language training?

                    YES   NO

    If YES, then the communicative response may be in the modality currently used in training. If previous speech/language training has been unsuccessful with all modalities, attempt simple gestures or symbols to start.

FIGURE 4-2. A completed checklist assessing the output modality to be used for teaching an alternate communicative response.

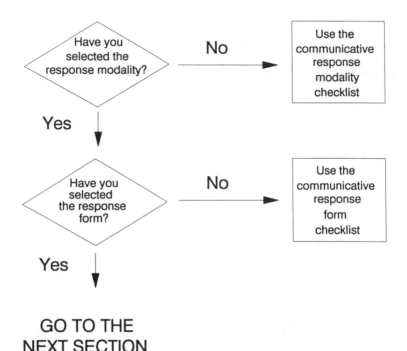

GO TO THE
NEXT SECTION

allowed to express a preference. The modality selected will also be affected by some of the issues described next in the section on "response form."

RESPONSE FORM

For the purposes of this training, an important consideration in selecting a particular communicative response is speed and ease of learning. Therefore an important question to ask about the form of the response is, *"Can it be easily taught?"* It is essential that the response be simple enough to be taught in the least amount of time. It may be, for example, that learning sign language has been identified as an important communication goal for this student. However, if learning a new sign has typically required more than a few weeks of training, then it is suggested that a simpler means of communicating be selected for initial training. Pointing to a picture of a desired activity or object, for example, can usually be taught in a relatively short period of time, and may therefore be considered as an alternative to sign language training for the purposes of reducing behavior problems.

As readers familiar with these issues will quickly note, a decision as to whether to use, for example, signs or pictorial forms as communicative responses can generate considerable controversy. Often professionals and caregivers have preferred communication systems that they incorporate into the language goals of most of the students with whom they work. Because of this, we have at times encountered resistance to using simpler forms of responses.

The rationale for beginning with a less complex response is that students can rapidly learn the behavior, and can quickly gain access to reinforcers (e.g., attention from others, favorite foods, activities). Because appropriate access to the stimuli that maintain problem behavior is the goal of functional communication training, it is important that this require as little effort as possible. Requiring a complex response (e.g., verbalizing a complete sentence, making a difficult sign) to obtain those reinforcers can lead to problems. Recently, one of our students illustrated the problems that teaching a complex response can generate.

TONY

Tony is a 14-year-old boy who lives in a group home and attends a segregated school in his neighborhood. Tony's teacher reported that he would frequently throw objects around the room and would at times scream and hit anyone who attempted to intervene. Although not always predictable, these tantrums frequently were elicited around those times when he appeared to want something (e.g., to go outside), but either couldn't have it or the teacher didn't know what he wanted.

Tony was capable of saying several words (e.g., "Mamma," "Home," and "Eat") but did not always use them appropriately and they were often hard to understand. Communication training with Tony involved "simultaneous communication," where the trainer would use both verbal cues and signs. And, although his signing vocabulary was more extensive than his verbal ability, his signs were also difficult for others to understand.

Following a number of assessment procedures, it was decided to teach him to request favorite objects appropriately (e.g., magazines) and activities (e.g., going for a walk). Both Tony's teacher and his speech therapist requested that he be taught to make the request verbally, because this was consistent with his communication goals. Functional communication training using verbal responses (i.e., having him say words or phrases such as "Outside?") was conducted daily for several months, with no measurable progress in his ability to verbalize his requests adequately, and no decreases in his tantrums. In fact, tantrums *increased*, especially around the time of communication training sessions. It appeared that asking him to verbalize the request was too much, and that he was trying to escape from the training sessions by being disruptive.

The recommendation was made to simplify the response requirements, and teach him simply to point to pictures of the things that he seemed to want. Within a few weeks, Tony was reliably requesting things he wanted by pointing to a variety of pictures without prompts, and concurrently, the frequency of his tantrums was greatly reduced.

This example points out some of the problems that can arise when the communicative response can't be taught quickly. Clearly, there are times when even the simplest response can be difficult to teach. For some individuals, even pointing to a picture can take a considerable amount of time to learn. However, it is always preferable to find a response that can be taught in the least amount of time. If desired, and once the response is being used successfully, training can begin on an alternate response that is more consistent with current communication goals. For example, in the example illustrated above, after Tony was successfully communicating through pictures, he was then encouraged to verbalize the requests at the same time.

If a student can verbally imitate, then the first suggestion for a mode of communication is through verbal means. Some students are verbal in that they are echolalic and/or perseverate verbally (e.g., repeat phrases or songs that they have heard). However, some of these students do not readily imitate words or phrases in more structured learning settings. If it appears that teaching the student to say a preferred word or phrase (e.g., "Help me") may be difficult, and may take more than a week to teach, then you may want to consider an alternative form of communication.

Two additional questions should be answered when selecting the type of communicative response to teach. The first of these questions, *"Can it be understood?"*, involves whether or not the response will be recognized by those in the prevailing environment, as well as those he or she may encounter in important settings in the future. For example, if a student can say "bathroom" verbally, but his or her articulation is such that those unfamiliar with him would not understand, then this will not be an effective communicative response. However, if the student points to the picture of a toilet, a person unfamiliar with the student and his or her programs could reasonably be expected to understand that the student is requesting to go to the bathroom.

We have frequently observed this problem with students who use signs as a means of communication. It is not uncommon to observe a student manipulating his or her hands in a particular manner so that only one or two others (e.g., a parent or teacher) can recognize its meaning. In fact, there is sometimes great pride taken by these individuals in their ability to understand the student when no one else can. From the student's perspective, however, this is a major problem. It means that only a small number of people can provide the student with his or her wants or needs. It terms of generalization and maintenance, therefore, the progress of the person will be limited to these individuals and the settings were they live or work. And, we have observed that success or failure in functional communication training can hinge on whether or not others understand the response. A student in one of our studies, Hal, illustrates this point quite clearly.

HAL

Hal was a 9-year-old boy who was attending a segregated school for students with developmental disabilities. Teachers reported that Hal frequently became upset at varying times during the day, typically in response to difficult requests and when he couldn't answer a question presented to him. He would violently slap his face and scream, ultimately falling to the floor. He had some verbal ability, although he would frequently talk rapidly and would slur his words.

As a first step, it was decided to teach him to say "I don't understand" in response to questions for which he didn't have an answer. After several weeks of this training, he would reliably and spontaneously use this communication strategy, and the frequency of his face slapping and screaming was substantially reduced. A follow-up observation of him several months later in a new classroom and with a different teacher, however, revealed that he was again slapping his face and screaming, and was rarely using the trained phrase.

Observing Hal with his new teacher, it was clear what was wrong. His teacher would ask a question such as "Hal, what's your address?" At times Hal would say, "I don't understand," but very quickly and unintelligibly. And, because the teacher didn't understand what he was saying, she did not provide him with sufficient prompts. After several interactions like this, Hal would eventually get upset, hit himself, and begin screaming. His teacher would respond by leaving him saying she would return when he calmed down. Therefore, not only did the teacher not respond to his statement, but she also appeared to be reinforcing his disruption by ending the task (negative reinforcement).

Our intervention involved working with Hal to slow down and better articulate the phrase "I don't understand." We did this without informing his teacher to see if she would respond appropriately to his phrase when it was intelligible. After our training, we again observed him in the classroom and found that he was more understandable, and that the teacher would now provide prompts for him (e.g., "Say, I live at 25 Smith Street") when he said he didn't understand. Additionally, his self-injury and screaming was again reduced. An additional follow-up observation 12 months later found Hal to be using the phrase and remaining well behaved in the classroom.

The next question to be asked is, *"Is it appropriate?"* In this context, it should be noted that different settings may call for different types of requests. For example, saying "Help me" may be appropriate when an individual is having difficulty dressing, but is not relevant in settings where the answer is known but the student wants a break from the task (an alternative response to be used in this setting might be "May I have a break?"). When beginning training, it is suggested that you start with one communicative response. *This response should be one that would be the most useful in the most settings, or most useful in the setting where there are the most problems.*

We use the Communicative Response "Form" Checklist to structure this assessment step. Once an initial response is selected for teaching to the student, the questions on the form are answered in order to anticipate any problems. For example, the responses from Lynn's form (see Figure 4-3) suggest that teaching her to request attention *verbally* would take more than a few weeks. Because a response using an alternate modality (e.g., pointing to pictures to get attention), might take much less time, this might be the way to intervene initially.

Additionally, the responses on the last two questions suggest that in her current setting, caregivers might ignore her requests for attention and may become annoyed. This is important information, but does not necessarily lead to an easy solution. Should you spend time trying to educate and train staff to respond appropriately, or should you change the response to one which will be acknowledged? We have been guided in these decisions by the issues described below.

Educational Relevance

One helpful guide that has assisted us in our efforts to select appropriate responses to teach is "the criterion of ultimate functioning" (Brown et al., 1976). This philosophy asserts that the skills you teach to students (in this case, the communicative response) should meet the criteria outlined below.

1. *The skill should be chronologically age-appropriate.* For example, teaching a 35-year-old man to say "Hug me" in order to gain attention from others (including strangers) would not be appropriate, and would probably be received negatively in most communities.

2. *The materials and activities needed to perform the skills should be present in the environment(s) in which the student currently lives or par-*

COMMUNICATIVE RESPONSE "FORM" CHECKLIST

Student's Name: _Lynn_   Date: _7/22/89_

Expected Response by Others: _Social attention_
(e.g., assistance, tangibles)

Communicative Response: _Verbally asking " May I help_
(Include form; e.g., verbal)   _you with that ?"_

Circle YES or NO for each of the questions below.

1. Is this response one that can be easily taught   YES   (NO)
   to the student (i.e., within a few days or
   weeks)?

2. Is this response one that could be understood   (YES)   NO
   by someone not familiar with the student?

3. Is this response appropriate for those   (YES)   NO
   situations in which most problem behaviors
   seem to occur?

4. Is this response one that will be responded   YES   (NO)
   to appropriately by other people?

5. If used appropriately, would other people   YES   (NO)
   not find this response annoying?

If you answered NO to any of the above questions, then a
different communicative response (i.e., form and/or modality)
should be considered.

FIGURE 4-3. A completed checklist used for assessing the form of the communicative response to be taught.

ticipates Necessary communication devices, for example, should be portable enough so that they can be taken to settings in which the student may wish to communicate.

3. _The skill should make the student more independent._ For example, when it is feasible, teaching students to request things by pointing to pictures rather than through signs (e.g., pointing to a picture of a glass of milk) may allow the student to obtain these things from individuals in their community who may not understand sign language. This would provide the student with more individuals with whom to communicate, and he or she would have to rely less on others with specific skills (e.g., staff members who can sign).

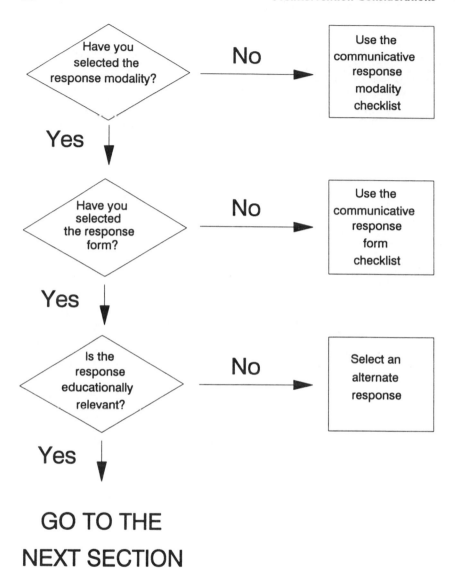

GO TO THE
NEXT SECTION

4. *The skill should prepare the student to function in community environments.* This is a critical component of skill selection. The communicative response being taught should be one that will be useful to students in their next placement. For example, in a regular school classroom, children without handicaps often obtain teacher attention by making statements such as "Am I doing good work?" or "Is this right?" These are the types of

attention-getting responses that should be taught to students who will be moving to regular school classrooms, as opposed to ones that might be viewed as annoying (e.g., "teacher, would you talk to me?").

Another way to view this issue relates to a concept referred to as "the natural communities of reinforcement" (Baer & Wolf, 1970). The goal here is to select and teach a communicative behavior that will elicit reinforcers in the prevailing environment. For example, if a student in a classroom enjoys the attention of others, then an important goal would be to teach him or her a behavior that will successfully gain attention from others *without* having to teach these other persons to respond appropriately. Using the example above, teachers typically respond to questions such as "Is this right?" by walking over to a student, and spending some time interacting with him or her (e.g., making statements such as, "Yes, that's very good!"). If important others in the environment will not respond as hoped to the students' communicative attempt, eventually the students will stop using the trained response, and will return to using inappropriate means of getting what they want.

Training Arrangements and Contexts

Once the communicative response has been selected, training should be conducted as often as possible. Ideally, training should be carried out throughout the day, especially when relevant, naturally occurring situations present themselves (Halle, 1988; Hart, 1985). For example, if you are teaching a student to make the sign for "Help" whenever assistance is needed, you may want to wait for a time when he or she normally requires help. For a student just entering school in the morning, putting his or her coat away may be difficult. The point at which he or she first walks in the building and takes the coat off would be an excellent time to prompt the sign, especially before he or she becomes upset. The student would be asking for help and subsequently receiving it at a time when he or she will most likely need assistance again.

Training throughout the day has been referred to as "distributed practice" (Gaylord–Ross & Holvoet, 1985; Mulligan, Lacy, & Guess, 1982; Sulzer–Azaroff & Mayer, 1986). In other words, students are allowed to engage in other activities between teaching trials. This is in contrast to "massed practice," which involves presenting teaching trials one after another, with limited interruptions. Most teaching occurs somewhere along a continuum from highly massed practice (very little time between teaching trials) to highly distributed practice (long delays between trials). There are several advantages to conducting training using an instructional format that

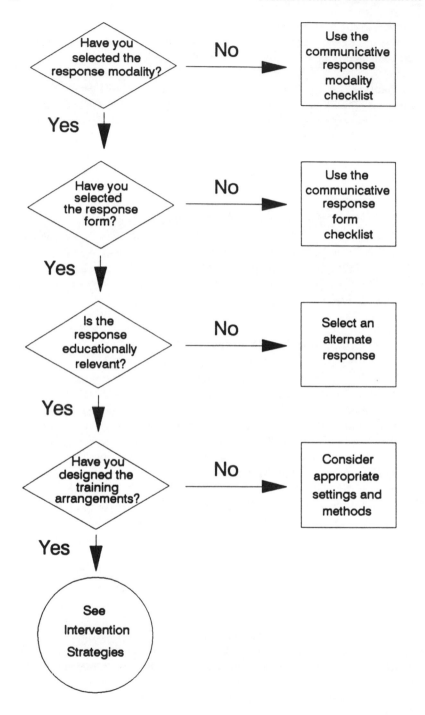

more closely conforms to the distributed-practice model. Because opportunities to make requests occur at varying times throughout the day, distributed practice more closely resembles these interactions. In addition, when compared to massed practice, such procedures have been demonstrated to be equal to or more effective in teaching skills to students (Mulligan et al., 1982).

Despite these advantages, initially using highly distributed practice with some students may be problematic. Because distributed practice as described above can involve fewer trials (although it doesn't have to), the opportunities to learn the skill may be sporadic. Acquisition may be slow, creating problems for students who may become disruptive to avoid such training situations. Additionally, training for staff in how to identify and use intermittent teaching opportunities may not be available in many settings (Alpert, 1984; Haring, Neetz, Lovinger, Peck, & Semmel, 1987; Schwartz, Anderson, & Halle, 1989).

Due to these limitations, *we have often begun training using more frequent teaching trials in a concentrated period of time.* We do this to ensure rapid acquisition, and because we are often faced with situations in which skilled trainers are available for a limited period of time during the day. For example, there may be one work supervisor who knows the learner best, and who is most capable of carrying out training. However, this person may be available for only 30 minutes each day to conduct teaching sessions. In these situations, we would set up training so that the supervisor could conduct a number of trials during that 30 minutes. Trials typically would be interspersed with breaks, opportunities to manipulate requested objects, or time for access to social interactions. *The environment is arranged to create opportunities for communication* (e.g., putting an obstacle in the path of a student's wheelchair and prompting him or her to ask for assistance). However, the initial sessions would not be carried out throughout the day until there was some initial success by the student in communication. The training arrangements might lie somewhere in the middle of the massed-practice/distributed-practice continuum. As soon as possible, however, training trials are interspersed throughout the student's day where appropriate.

The settings or contexts in which such teaching takes place can also be viewed on a continuum from highly artificial contexts (e.g., teaching social interactions with peers in a therapist's office) to more natural contexts (e.g., teaching social interactions with peers at a party). *The "naturalness" of the setting depends largely on where you want the student to use the new communicative response.* Generalization and maintenance of intervention effects may be facilitated by using the criterion environment (i.e., where you want the student to communicate) as the training environment. With the typical model of teaching skills in a separate setting (e.g., in the speech therapist's office), once the response is learned you need to encourage the performance of that behavior in settings where you want it to occur (e.g., in the cafeteria). *By beginning training in the natural or criterion setting, extensive programming for generalization is not necessary because it will be occurring where you want it to occur. In addition, obstacles to maintenance can be immediately identified when teaching in the criterion environment* (e.g., are the consequences being provided in that setting going to maintain the new response?) (Halle, 1988).

Unlike the qualifications for training arrangements outlined above, *we have not found it necessary to use artificial contexts to conduct training.* Except in cases where the natural setting may need to be modified for safety reasons, training should always be conducted where you want the student to use the new communicative response (Berkman & Meyer, 1988).

One case we worked with involved teaching communication to a student with extremely severe self-injurious behavior. Staff members were concerned that the student might seriously hurt himself if they attempted training in the typical workshop setting (he would hit his head on the corners of tables). They noted that he was relatively free of self-injury when he was alone in his room, and this was assumed to be due to the lack of demands and the lack of resemblance to work settings. What was recommended was to replicate part of his room in the workshop. His favorite chair was brought into the workshop room and was placed away from the worktable. He was allowed to sit in this chair, and for several weeks no demands were placed on him while he sat in this chair. Once he was well behaved in the workshop in his chair, functional communication training was initiated. In this case, the training situation was modified to lessen the risk of injury. However, this type of extensive modification of the environment is rarely needed, and such changes should be made only as a last resort.

Figure 4-4 illustrates the continua for training arrangements and training contexts just discussed, and their relationship to generalization and maintenance. *To maximize generalization and maintenance, training efforts should focus on more distributed practice in natural settings or contexts.* Again, although initial acquisition may require more massed practice, the goal should always be toward distributing trials throughout a student's day.

Summary

This section discussed general issues related to functional communication training including, how to decide to intervene, selecting the communicative response, and selecting the teaching setting. Presented here were general guidelines for making many of these decisions. These guidelines are outlined

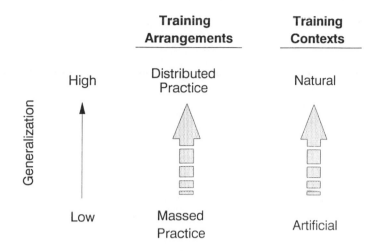

FIGURE 4-4. An illustration of the training arrangements and contexts and their potential impact on stimulus and response generalization.

for readers in the flow charts presented throughout this chapter. In what follows, functional communication training will be described in more detail, with more specific recommendations on how to conduct training. Again, however, it must be stressed that these procedures will probably need to be modified to be relevant to the person with whom you are working, and for the setting where the teaching will take place.

5

Intervention Strategies

"We want to make good time, but for us now this is measured
with emphasis on 'good' rather than 'time' and when you make
that shift in emphasis the whole approach changes."

(PIRSIG, 1974, p. 5)

There are two primary components to functional communication training:
The students are taught a response that serves the same function as their
challenging behavior and, at the same time, there is an attempt to make the
problem behavior nonfunctional. The first component is accomplished with
communication training, and the second is achieved through response-independent consequences for problem behavior. These aspects of intervention
are applied simultaneously, and are essential to its success. What follows is
a discussion and description of these two aspects of functional communication training. We start with a discussion of the skills-training aspect of this
intervention, because it has been well studied, and because we believe it is
central to the effectiveness of this intervention approach.

A multiphase prompting and prompt-fading procedure is used to teach
the new communicative response. Prompts are introduced as necessary, then
faded as quickly as possible. To illustrate initial response training, examples
are presented from individuals whom we have taught such things as requests
for assistance on tasks or a break from work, requests for social attention,
requests for tangibles, and requests for sensory feedback. And, because this
training never occurs outside of the social and political contexts in which
the person lives, included are aspects of the intervention that are not typically
discussed in chapters or journal articles focused on intervention. Intervention for severe behavior problems is a complex task, often involving change
at many levels (e.g., administrative, social, personal). Therefore, issues
addressing concerns such as the controversy over interventions using aver-

sive stimuli, staffing problems, and opposition by administrators will be examined where relevant.

Teaching Requests for Assistance/Escape

One of the more unpleasant responsibilities required of any educator is working with an individual who actively or passively resists teaching. Some learners "negatively resist" attempts to teach important skills (e.g., student screams and kicks), others "positively resist" (e.g., student laughs and giggles instead of working), and still others "passively resist" (e.g., student does not look at materials, makes no response). When a student kicks, screams, and rips up work materials whenever they are presented, or passively ignores efforts to get him or her to attend to a task, teaching becomes a major challenge and learning becomes highly unlikely.

One procedure we have used for these types of problems is to teach the student to request assistance (e.g., "Help me") or a brief "break" from work. Often the problem behaviors exhibited by students appear to be attempts to avoid or escape from unpleasant situations. It makes sense, then, that if the student is taught to request assistance appropriately *and receives it*, the task

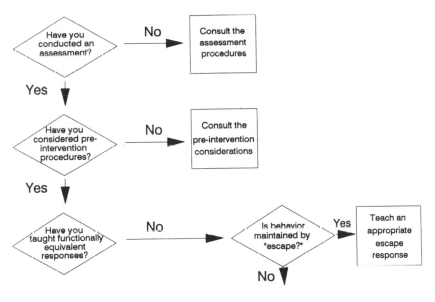

GO TO THE
NEXT SECTION

will seem easier and problem behaviors should be reduced. Similarly, if a student has been working for some time on a task and is allowed to ask for a break *and receives it,* this student's problem behavior should also be reduced. What follows is a description of the training procedures we have used to teach students to request assistance or breaks from work appropriately and spontaneously. Work with one man will be used to illustrate these procedures.

Bill

Recently, a young man (Bill) was brought to our attention because he was engaging in severe aggression (punching and grabbing others), self-injurious behavior (hand and arm biting), and other disruptive behaviors (throwing work materials, knocking over tables and chairs). Bill was 32 years old at the time of the referral, and had lived most of his life in a large institution. He had recently moved from the institution to a group home and was attending a vocational education program through a local agency.

The vocational program was concerned because Bill was making only minimal progress, and would occasionally hurt staff members seriously. An analysis of ABC charts along with administrations of the MAS indicated that his aggression and self-injury may have been maintained by both escape from demands, and access to tangibles (e.g., favorite foods). It was decided to begin by teaching him the sign for "break" and allowing him to take time away from work if he asked. A request to leave work was selected, as opposed to a request for tangibles, because the work demands appeared to elicit the most frequent and severe outbursts. A request for a break was chosen over a request for assistance because he had no difficulty completing the work (i.e., it wasn't difficult), and because it was appropriate at a job site to request a period of time away from work.

Training began in the vocational setting because this was where he had been referred and where most of the problems occurred. The intervention sessions were carried out approximately 30 minutes per day. This was the amount of time the agency could spare for one-to-one intervention. We assessed that he would tolerate approximately 60 seconds of work before he would get upset, so we planned to require him to work for 10–15 seconds prior to prompting him to sign. This was an effort to prevent him from becoming upset and hurting staff or himself.

For the first sessions, work was placed in front of Bill as it normally would be and, after the 10–15 seconds of his working, (1) the trainer pulled back the materials, (2) the trainer said "Sign Break," (3) the trainer physically prompted him to sign "Break," and (4) the trainer led Bill to a corner of the room for a 1–2-minute break. Table 5-1 illustrates these training steps.

TABLE 5-1. Prompt fading steps for teaching sign for a "break" from work

Phase	Prompt Level 1	Prompt Level 2	Prompt Level 3	Prompt Level 4	Student Response	Trainer Response
I	Vocational setting	Task is removed	Trainer says, "Sign Break"	Trainer physically prompts sign for "Break"	Signs "Break"	Allows students to spend time away from work
II	Vocational setting	Task is removed	Trainer says, "Sign Break"		Signs "Break"	Allows students to spend time away from work
III	Vocational setting	Task is removed			Signs "Break"	Allows students to spend time away from work
IV	Vocational setting				Signs "Break"	Allows students to spend time away from work

Bill's response to our initial training efforts was characteristic of many individuals with whom we have worked. He was fine during the prompting, and while he was going on the break. However, when we attempted to bring him back to work, he resisted. Occasionally he would hit the trainer, or passively resist efforts to get him back to the worktable. During these times he was firmly led back to work in a neutral manner, with no reprimands or lengthy explanations. This resistance quickly abated over several sessions. It appeared as if Bill learned that if he went right back to work, he could escape it within a short amount of time.

As Table 5-1 describes, we began pulling back our prompts by first fading the physical prompt. We did this by going from a full physical prompt to partial prompts (e.g., just touching his hand), to gestural prompts (e.g., motioning to prompt his hands), to, finally, only the verbal prompt "Say, Break." Throughout his training we relied heavily on delayed prompting (Halle, Baer, Spradlin, 1981; Schwartz et al., 1989). After several trials, we would intersperse a trial with a delayed prompt (i.e., we waited approximately 5 seconds), to see if Bill would respond without the next level of prompt. For example, if he had been responding to just a touch of his hand to sign, we would make a gesture as if we were going to prompt him, and then wait 5 seconds. If he made the sign for "Break," then we would let him go on the break.

We did not wait until responding was extremely stable to move on to the next level of prompting. In other words, he did not have to be correctly responding to say, 9 out of 10 prompts for 2 weeks for us to move to the next step. We would attempt to move to the next step if he was successful at a step for 3 to 5 consecutive responses. We did this in order to prevent him from becoming too reliant on prompts to respond.

Training progressed quickly over several weeks to the point where he would sign for a break with only the act of pulling back the work as a prompt (see Prompt Level 2 in Table 5-1). This too was faded, and within 3 months he was requesting a break without any cues by the trainer. As is typical in our training, his behavior improved most dramatically as soon as he began to make requests without prompts.

Once successful, intervention continued by introducing new signs (e.g., food, music, work), reintroducing work demands, expanding the settings in which his signs were encouraged to include his whole day, and introducing new staff into the training program. These latter steps were introduced systematically, to avoid having him become disruptive. Nine months after initial intervention, the number of episodes of aggression and self-injury was significantly decreased, he was using a large number of signs spontaneously throughout the day, and he was working at a level that exceeded his preintervention performance.

The previous example illustrated a number of steps that are common to most of our intervention efforts. For example, proper fading of prompts is crucial. It should occur quickly enough to prevent prompt dependency, but not so fast that it results in too many errors by the student and, subsequently results in increased problem behavior. This balance is difficult to quantify because it varies from student to student. Our rule of thumb has been to use the student's behavior as a guide. If we find that training is beginning to result in some disruption by the student, then we will go back a step (i.e., provide a higher level of prompt). Again, especially for students with escape-maintained problem behavior, it is important that training not become another aversive demand.

Selecting the Training Setting

The prompting efforts just illustrated are consistent with discussion in the Assessment chapter on creating situations with low rates of problem behavior. For all training efforts *there is an attempt to set up the teaching situation so that the student is engaging in the fewest number problem behaviors possible.* An errorless learning procedure is attempted so that stimuli such as task demands, amount of teacher attention, and tangibles are faded in and/or faded out to reduce the baseline levels of challenging behavior (Touchette, 1968; Weeks & Gaylord–Ross, 1981). The purpose of these efforts is to reduce the disruption during teaching sessions, and to lower the possible risk to the student and to others.

In addition to these considerations, the setting for training assistance seeking or requests for a break should be relevant to the request. If problem behaviors occur in certain demand situations (e.g., following requests to make their beds or during difficult tabletop tasks), then training should take place in that setting (i.e., the bedroom or at a table in the classroom, respectively). In the example just described, training for Bill was conducted at his workshop, with the materials on which he was being asked to work. *It is important to avoid training in settings that are very different from the places you wish the student to use the communicative response.* For example, do not train in a "therapy" room if you want a student to request a break from work; training should occur in the actual work setting.

When teaching a request for a break from work, the setting that will serve as a break area will need to be selected. This varies with the student you are working with and the setting where training is carried out. Some situations call for keeping the student at the desk where work is carried out and just removing the work materials. In other cases, a separate desk may be designated as the break desk, or an area of the room can be used. In any case, several considerations should be kept in mind. First, does the setting to be used approximate what a break would look like in this setting if your student did not have a disability? For example, try not to use the floor if at all possible. Even though the student may prefer to sit on the floor, avoid this as a break because it will have to be faded out later (i.e., you will need to begin to move him or her to a chair or couch to have the break look more appropriate).

Bill's training involved the use of signs to request a break from work. A second student, Mary Ann, illustrates how we carry out functional communication training with someone who has not been successful in using any formal communication method. However, because there were a number of controversial components to this program, a detailed description of Mary Ann's intervention history and the background on this case are included before the details of functional communication training with her are discussed.

Mary Ann

Mary Ann was 33 years old at the time of our first contact. She had an extensive history of severe and frequent self-injurious head hitting, and had lived in a large institutional setting for most of her life. Mary Ann had severe sensory impairments (deaf and blind) and was required to be in full arm restraints during the day to prevent further injury to herself. At least one member of the staff at the institution was very close to Mary Ann, having worked with her for over 10 years.

Our involvement began with a request to conduct a review of Mary Ann's behavior management program. The request centered around a contingent electric shock program, and whether this program should be continued as an intervention for Mary Ann's self-injurious behavior. The records were reviewed, discussions with staff were conducted, and observations of Mary Ann during several activities were made.

Following is a brief description of Mary Ann's intervention history:

(1) Psychotropic medication—Thorazine, Haldol, Mellaril, Valium
(2) Overcorrection
(3) Required relaxation
(4) Contingent water mist
(5) Contingent restraint removal
(6) Contingent lemon juice
(7) Contingent Listerine
(8) Contingent ice

All of the above procedures (except medication) were attempted for relatively brief periods of time (i.e., from several minutes to several months), and all were abandoned because of their apparent lack of effectiveness with Mary Ann's self-injurious behavior. More recently, Mary Ann participated in a series of sessions, the goal of which was to assess the effectiveness of a contingent electric shock program. She was involved in 44 brief treatment sessions, which lasted a total of approximately 2 hours. During that time, Mary Ann received approximately 1,200 shocks for self-injury. These trials were discontinued, and a review of the program was recommended.

In making recommendations on the use of this program, the pros and cons were evaluated. What follows is a list of both the advantages and the disadvantages of reinstating the contingent electric shock program. Every effort was made to solicit objective and subjective input from all persons concerned.

ADVANTAGES

Past Failed Programs. Many of the procedures using aversive stimuli documented in the contemporary research literature had been attempted with Mary Ann in the past (e.g., contingently applied overcorrection, water mist, lemon juice). Clinically effective results with these procedures were limited.

Documentation. Contingent electric shock is a well-documented intervention procedure for self-injurious behavior (Favell et al., 1982). In those cases where it has been successful, this procedure has resulted in initial dramatic reductions in these behaviors.

Supervision. The shock program and the device to be used had been designed and would have been supervised by a professional experienced in the use of contingent electric shock.

Staff Concerns. The staff involved with Mary Ann's program had gone to extraordinary lengths to implement and document its work with procedures involving aversive stimuli. This effort was highly commendable, and reflected the care and concern all had shown for Mary Ann's welfare. Many of these individuals had worked with Mary Ann for several years and were concerned with her continued lack of progress. Many of the professional and paraprofessional staff members who had direct contact with Mary Ann expressed a desire to see the contingent electric shock program reinstated. They felt that the initial trials produced encouraging changes in Mary Ann's self-injurious behavior.

Improvements in the Shock Device. Based on discussions with the consultant supervising the shock trials and an examination and a personal test of the device, the new version of the device that was being recommended for use seemed to be capable of more consistent introduction of electric shock. There may have been less of a chance that participants would receive shocks for behaviors other than head hitting. In addition, the consultant indicated that the shock pack would be placed on Mary Ann's leg instead of her arm to reduce the likelihood of her removing it.

DISADVANTAGES

Ethical Concerns. Clearly, there is no consensus on the appropriate use of interventions using extremely aversive stimuli with individuals exhibiting severe developmental disabilities. There are those who would argue that any use of a procedure such as contingent electric shock is unwarranted and unethical. Among the reasons cited include the inability to obtain informed consent from the participant, and the human concern of deliberately producing pain in another person. The review was not designed to resolve such ethical dilemmas. However, it was important to note that contingent electric shock is a controversial procedure, and one must consider this fact when evaluating whether it should be used.

Previous Initial Results. One of the major disadvantages in reinstating the contingent electric shock program concerned the lack of immediate and dramatic results from the trials. The data suggested that Mary Ann's hits to her head were reduced by approximately 50% and hits above threshold (i.e., hits severe enough to receive shocks) were reduced by approximately 70% with the contingent electric shock program, compared to nontreated observations. Although these represent significant reductions in her self-injury, the reductions were not consistent with previous work using contingent electric shock. When previous attempts to reduce similar behaviors with electric shock had been successful, the reductions were on the order of 90%—100% within the first few trials (Carr & Lovaas, 1983; Favell et al., 1982; Romanczyk, Kistner, & Plienis, 1982). The following are quotes from one review (Carr & Lovaas, 1983) of the treatment literature using electric shock:

> In general, unless there is a marked decrease in the rate of self-injurious behavior in at least one situation in the presence of at least one therapist following 5–10 shocks, the procedure will probably fail and should be discontinued. (p. 228)

> Large amounts of punishment should be avoided, otherwise adaptation to the shock is likely to occur. Typically, only a few shocks are needed to produce initial suppression and maintain that effect. (p. 232)

These immediate and dramatic reductions are to be expected when an extremely aversive stimulus such as electric shock is employed. The results with Mary Ann were not consistent with other documented successes in the research literature or expert recommendations.

Lack of Improving Trends. In addition to expecting rapid suppression of self-injurious behavior when using contingent electric shock, the trend of these results should have pointed to an improving pattern of behavior. In other words, self-injury should continue to decline in frequency and approach extremely low levels within a short period of time. However, this declining trend in self-injury was not evident in Mary Ann's data. The data suggested that her self-injurious hits were relatively stable across time. Again, these results were not consistent with previous successful intervention efforts using contingent electric shock (Carr & Lovaas, 1983; Favell et al., 1982; Romanczyk et al., 1982). In addition, the relatively high number of shocks administered (over 1,200 during approximately 2 hours of treatment) were of clinical concern, because habituation to the shock is likely under these conditions.

Avoiding Shock. It was clear from observing the videotapes of the shock sessions that Mary Ann quickly (in a matter of seconds) learned to avoid receiving shocks. In at least one session, her hits to her head (followed by shock) were modified to hits to her chin (which did not receive shocks). On another occasion, she was able to position her head in such a way that again made the device ineffective. There was a concern that she would be able to discriminate those conditions under which she would not get shocked, thereby negating the effects of the program. For example, the device is not effective if the participant takes off the head piece. It was possible that Mary Ann would learn this, and the staff would be left with further modifications on the device to keep the device on her head. Additionally, such self-injurious behaviors as scratches to her legs were not detected by the current device, and could increase.

Limitations of the Device. A major limitation of the shock device as designed was that it couldn't deliver the electric shock following each instance of Mary Ann's self-injurious hits. Because Mary Ann engaged in such rapid self-injury (i.e., over 200 hits per minute), the delay built into the device for safety reasons resulted in her being able to hit herself several times without being shocked. This pattern of responding could have resulted in an intermittent schedule of punishment, a situation that is not ideal for complete response suppression (Luiselli & Townsend, 1980). In fact, there was a concern with this schedule that self-injurious behavior would be maintained, albeit at a lower rate than baseline (this pattern appears to have been reflected in the data collected).

This device is only designed to be used with the headpiece for head banging. Other forms of self-injury are not targeted by the self-activated part of this device. Also, the device cannot differentiate a self-inflicted hit from an accidental head bump, a fall, or a push by another person. In addition, the electrode is held on with velcro, making it possible to remove the electrode. This results in one more problem (similar to using restraints), trying to find ways to keep the electrode on the individual.

Also, by not involving staff directly in the presentation of the shock (because it is self-activated), the clinical judgment and responsibility is removed from well-trained individuals familiar with the individual. And, even if the self-activated part of the device is not used, using a remote device puts undesirable distance between the targeted individual and the educator/clinician.

Aside from general concerns about using contingent electric shock, there is also a concern when using experimental devices. At the time of the review, there had been no controlled, published accounts of the successful use of this device with any behavior problem. And, even anecdotal reports of its use had rarely reported successful fading of the device.

Long-term Acceptability. Although there were some limited provisions made for fading out the use of the shock device, research has shown that such an intervention may be a lifelong effort. For example, a recent study (Foxx, McMorrow, Bittle, & Bechtel, 1986) demonstrated the ability of contingent electric shock to reduce severe aggression in one man. However, a follow-up of this case 15 months postintervention showed that periodic shocks were still necessary. The concern here was that staff members would be reluctant to fade the shock program. It was also expected that they would avoid taking Mary Ann out of the institution and into the local community if it were apparent to community members that she were receiving electric shocks.

Functional Analysis. Although it was noted in some of the reports that Mary Ann's motivation for self-injury may have involved escape (i.e., she is attempting to escape or avoid unpleasant situations through her self-injury), no apparent provisions were made in the plan to teach her an alternative response (e.g., to communicate this request). There was a concern that even if the shock program significantly reduced Mary Ann's self-injury, the "crisis" would be over, and limited effort would be spent teaching her these alternatives.

Least Restrictive Alternative. At the time the original succession of programs using aversive stimuli were initiated (over 6 years prior to this review), many of the then-documented alternatives had been explored as options for Mary Ann's severe self-injurious behavior. However, in light of the research conducted since that time, there were a number of less restrictive procedures that had not been attempted with Mary Ann.

RECOMMENDATIONS AND PROGRAM SUGGESTIONS

It was recommended that the electric shock program *not* be reinstated. The disadvantages of reinstating this program appeared to far outweigh the advantages, when all aspects of Mary Ann's habilitation goals were considered. This recommendation was based on the information presented above, especially the apparent lack of effective results from the experimental trials and the predicted problems with future attempts to use contingent electric shock with Mary Ann.

This recommendation was also based on the assumption that the technology of intervention using techniques without aversive stimuli had advanced considerably in the time since the first restrictive intervention was attempted, and that Mary Ann could benefit from such procedures. Given all of this information, Mary Ann did not appear to be a good candidate for using contingent electric shock.

It was further recommended that attempts be made to teach Mary Ann to request certain preferred reinforcers (e.g., walks, swimming, music, certain foods, time alone). Such an intervention had proven to be an effective behavior reduction technique with other individuals with severe handicaps who were exhibiting severe behavior problems.

The circumstances surrounding Mary Ann and the interventions for her self-injurious behavior posed some important obstacles that would be helpful to discuss. First, attempting to introduce functional communication training at this point was anticipated to result in some opposition. Most of the staff members and many of the clinicians supported the continuation of the electric shock program, and were of the opinion that all less restrictive alternatives had been tried and had failed. As mentioned previously, there was an assumption that "less restrictive equaled less effective," therefore no less restrictive procedure could be effective if something as intrusive as electric shock was producing minor positive effects. Second, because of the frequency and intensity of her self-injury, having her use her hands to communicate would be problematic. It was anticipated that any effort to release her hands during training would result in her hitting herself. Third, there were severe limitations in staff time to conduct the program and as well as the availability of choice in most aspects of her daily life. For example, because meals were prepared elsewhere, there were almost no options for Mary Ann to select preferred foods. Similarly, staff were reluctant to take her into the local community because of the presence of her restraints.

Despite these and other obstacles, it was decided to attempt functional communication training with this woman. Given the level of commitment by the staff for previous programs, it was hoped that if they "bought into the program," they could teach Mary Ann to communicate basic needs and wants, and that her self-injury could subsequently be reduced. What follows is a synopsis of the intervention plan that was presented to staff at the facility where Mary Ann lived.

REPORT TO STAFF

Initial assessment of Mary Ann's self-injurious behaviors seems to indicate that they are influenced by more than one variable. However, the most common reason why she engages in this behavior appears to be to escape or avoid unpleasant or demanding situations. There are times when she also hits herself to get favorite foods and drinks, and may hit herself occasionally to gain attention. In addition, some of the lighter hits to her head may serve a self-stimulatory function. However, she appears to use her self-injury most frequently to escape or avoid undesirable activities. Therefore, we will begin by teaching her one alternative escape response.

Training will begin by getting Mary Ann to hand you a token with the words "I want my restraints" written on it. The token should be rounded and made of a soft material so that she will not hurt herself if she hits her head with it. Also, you should pick a token that has several varieties, to plan for future additions to her communicative repertoire. This response was chosen because (1) Mary Ann appears to enjoy her restraints, (2) putting on her restraints signals the end of most demands and, (3) this is a good way for her to begin to communicate her desire to end unpleasant situations. Using a token is recommended because it will facilitate communication. Messages can be written on the token so that she can tell persons not familiar with her program what she wants.

This training should probably be carried out in her room to start, taking the training to other settings once she is successfully using the token. Her room seems appropriate because she often has her restraints removed here, and her favorite chair is in her room.

1. Training should begin by having Mary Ann stand up from her chair and removing one of her arms from the restraint (her unrestrained arm should be held or "shadowed" so that she does not harm herself).

2. The token should be placed in her hand. If she drops it, pick it up and put it back into her unrestrained hand.

3. Physically and verbally prompt her to give you back the token. Because she may have some residual hearing, verbal prompts may be useful. Initially, you may need to take the token from her. Table 5-2 illustrates the prompt fading steps used with Mary Ann.

4. Once the token is given back to you, place her restraint back on her arm. Let her sit or stand (whichever she seems to prefer) for 1–2 minutes with her restraint on before starting again.

5. Remove the restraint, and repeat the prompting steps 1–4. Sessions should last no more than 30 minutes. Be careful not to go too long; otherwise she might find the session aversive and try to escape by hitting herself.

6. Once she successfully hands you the token with the prompts 3–5 times in a row, begin to fade the prompts. Begin by only touching her hand after you place the token in it, then move to a touch, removing your hand (so that she has to reach out to give it to you) (see Table 5-2).

7. If she succeeds in handing you the token after she is given it without physical or verbal prompts, then fade out your holding her unrestrained arm. Thus, the next step is to get to the point where you take off the restraint and, not restraining her arm, give her the token and she returns it. Once she successfully completes this step 3–5 times in a row, begin to introduce new staff members to the program. The first teacher should instruct other staff on how to conduct the program as described above. Once a staff person has Mary Ann successfully responding at the level above 3–5 times in a row, additional staff members can be introduced.

TABLE 5-2. Prompt fading steps for teaching requests for restraints

Phase	Prompt Level 1	Prompt Level 2	Prompt Level 3	Prompt Level 4	Student Response	Trainer Response
I	Restraints are removed	Token is handed to student	Touch student's hand	Hand over hand, places token in trainer's hand	Gives token to trainer	Replaces restraints on student
II	Restraints are removed	Token is handed to student	Touch student's hand		Gives token to trainer	Replaces restraints on student
III	Restraints are removed	Token is handed to student			Gives token to trainer	Replaces restraints on student
IV	Restraints are removed	Student is carrying token			Gives token to trainer	Replaces restraints on student

8. Once several new staffers have been successful, begin the next level of prompt fading by removing both arms from restraints and proceeding through the training steps as above.

Reacting to Her Self-injury. At no time should anyone talk to Mary Ann about her self-injury. For example, if she hits herself hard, do not tell her to use lighter taps. Also, if she digs her nails into you, try not to respond other than protecting yourself (i.e., do not make comments such as, "Please don't do that!"). Additionally, try not to end a session because she is hitting herself. Try to keep the schedule consistent. This is extremely important! We do not want to change the way we are reacting to her based on her problem behavior.

Data Collection. Data collection should include the number of training trials (i.e., how many times you give her the token), the number of successful trials (i.e., how many times she hands you the token), the best response she displays for that session, and the data on her self-injury (see Figure 5-1). Copies of the data sheet provided should be made to keep records of all

FUNCTIONAL COMMUNICATION TRAINING
DATA SHEET

Student's Name: __Mary Ann__   Date: _7/27/88_

Training days [date]	Number of training trials attempted	Number of successful trials	Best response	Frequency of problem behavior
7/27/88	‖‖ ‖	‖	phys. prompt	20
7/28/88	‖‖	‖‖	touch to arm	5
7/29/88	‖‖	‖	touch to arm	5
7/29/88	‖‖	‖‖‖	touch to arm	2

FIGURE 5-1. A typical data sheet used during functional communication training. The "best response" is recorded to facilitate the rapid progress of training steps.

sessions. Collecting data in this way will give us information on her percentage of correct responses, the frequency of her self-injury, and a way to follow her "best responses." Because we want to move quickly through the prompt fading stages, knowing that she engaged in one or two advanced steps may help us make decisions about moving ahead.

Mary Ann's progress through the program described above was slow. Although during many of the sessions she appeared happy, and *the frequency of her self-injury was only 10%-20% of its pretreatment levels* (which exceeded the results of the contingent electric shock program), she was having difficulty learning the communicative response. Changing from the tokens to more iconic objects (e.g., a piece of leather to represent a request for her restraints, a small cup to represent a request for a drink, a toy chair to represent a request to sit down) facilitated this learning. This change (which occurred almost 10 months into the program) and her improved performance coincided with reports that she was spending some entire days without her restraints. Four months later, staffers were observing Mary Ann's spontaneous use of the communicative objects and reported that weeks of her not hitting herself were now continuous. As of this writing, *she has gone over 18 months without any restraints, with no injury to herself, and the physician's order for restraints has been removed from her record for the first time in recent memory.* Staff also report increased contact with the community and her participation in more and varied activities throughout the day.

Mary Ann's case is important for several reasons. First, it illustrates that *useful communication skills can be taught to individuals with profound disabilities.* Second, although we observed an immediate reduction in Mary Ann's self-injury during training sessions that was equal to or better than other more aversive intervention efforts (including the contingent electric shock), we considered the program to be a failure until the effects generalized to nonintervention settings. This was in contrast with previous efforts in which reductions in Mary Ann's self-injury during intervention sessions alone were considered a success. In this case, functional communication training produced a quick suppression of self-injury; however, generalization required almost a year of effort.

In addition, this example provides an instance of how some of the models we have come to adopt for introducing interventions may be inappropriate. Readers may recall the discussion in the Introduction which focused on the "least restrictive alternative" and the "rapid suppression" philosophies of intervention. In Mary Ann's case, staff persons had presumably run through all of the "less restrictive alternatives," and were attempting some of the most restrictive interventions (e.g., contingent electric shock). For many of those involved, it was thought that going back to a less restrictive intervention, such as functional communication training, could not possibly be effective because of the assumption that "less restrictive equals less effective." At least for Mary Ann the reverse of this assumption was true—*the less restrictive alternative was more effective than the more restrictive alternative*. This case suggests that an intervention that is less restrictive may still be successful, even after more restrictive interventions have been attempted and have failed.

Using a symbolic form of communication such as Mary Ann's tokens is only one way to intervene when verbal language and sign language training have not been successful (Reichle & Karlan, 1985). Other augmentative systems are available, and efforts with one young boy using pictures as communication will now be discussed to illustrate these efforts. Dave's program also describes more specifically how criteria are used to move from one training step to the next.

Dave

Dave was 7 years old at the time of intervention, and had been referred because of frequent and chronic self-injury and tantrums. Dave would bite his hand, slap his face, scream, and fall to the floor numerous times throughout the day. He was well liked by his teachers. His communication skills were limited to pointing to what he wanted. He rarely played or socialized with other children, and spent large portions of his free time by himself.

Assessments involving analogue observations and the MAS suggested that escape from unpleasant situations was an important influence on his problem behaviors. This was consistent with teacher reports and reports from his family that he would most likely get upset when asked to work.

It was decided that because many of the tasks he was working on seemed difficult for him, teaching him to communicate for assistance would be appropriate in most of these situations. If he regularly received help on tasks, they should seem easier, and he may not want to escape them so frequently. A picture of a teacher helping a student was created for this purpose, along with pictures of other activities he may want later on in training. What follows are the instructions given to Dave's teachers on how to teach him to point to this picture when he needed assistance.

DAVE'S PROGRAM

We will use pointing to a picture of a teacher helping a student as a request for assistance. The first step in training involves prompting Dave to point to the appropriate picture in the selected setting. Begin with only one picture on the table if Dave does not readily the discriminate pictures.

This step involves full physical prompts. With task materials on the table, (1) have Dave attempt some small piece of fairly difficult work, (2) pull back the work materials, (3) say to Dave "Point to help," and (4) physically guide his finger to the picture. When Dave points to the picture say something like "Oh, you want help" and then provide an appropriate prompt.

Criterion. Repeat the training steps outlined above until Dave successfully points to the picture of "help" with prompts approximately 3–5 times in a row.

Once Dave completes this step, begin to *fade out the physical prompts.* This can be done by bringing Dave's hand only part of the way to the picture and/or by delaying the prompt for a few seconds. Continue to say "Point to help" but systematically reduce the amount of physical guidance you provide. For example, we taught one student to point to the picture of a help by using *delayed prompting.* This involved, (1) having the student complete some small piece of work, (2) pulling back the work materials, (3) saying "Point to help," and (4) waiting several seconds (2–5) before physically guiding his finger to the picture. This was highly successful in assisting the student in pointing to the picture with only our verbal prompts.

Criterion. Once Dave correctly points to the picture of assistance with only the verbal prompt approximately 3–5 times in a row, proceed to the next step of training.

This step involves fading out the verbal prompt, "Point to help." We accomplished this by, (1) having Dave complete some small piece of work, (2) pulling back the work materials, and (3) waiting several seconds before we said to Dave "Point to help." Again, this should be successful in having Dave point to the picture with only the pulling back of the work materials as the prompt.

Criterion. Once Dave correctly points to the picture of assistance approximately 3–5 times in a row with only the pulling back of the work material as a prompt, proceed to the next step.

This step involves fading out all teacher prompts. We accomplish this by intermittently pulling back the work materials, waiting for Dave to use the trained communicative response. This resembles the delayed prompt procedure described above, in that the prompt (pulling back materials) is delayed until Dave begins to "spontaneously" request help.

Criterion. Once Dave correctly points to the picture of assistance approximately 3–5 times in a row without teacher prompts, proceed to the next step.

This is the final step in initial response training, and involves the gradual reintroduction of work requirements into the training setting. Many times when this type of training is successful, students will begin to request assistance even for tasks that previously were completed without effort. It is difficult to define precisely how the work requirements in these cases should be reintroduced and how fast this should be accomplished. This training step will require the judgment of all staff involved with the program.

Several assumptions, however, have guided our past efforts during this point in training. First, *we have tried to make this stage "errorless."* In other words, because the task demands have traditionally predicted the presence of problem behavior in students with escape-maintained behavior, introducing work that is very difficult too soon might result in dramatic increases in problem behavior. Therefore, we have typically broken down the tasks to be introduced into smaller, more easily accomplished steps, that can be introduced one at a time.

Our second assumption, however, has been *not to wait too long to reintroduce new work.* As you could see in the criteria we set up for each training step, we only wait until the student responds correctly 3–5 times in a row before we move to the next step. Traditionally, teachers have been instructed to wait until students respond correctly for several weeks before changing training steps. We have found that waiting this long appears to make the process of changing steps more difficult. Thus, our general guideline has been to reintroduce new work quickly, but to break up the new work into smaller segments.

This, of course, is always guided by the reaction of the student. If you introduce a small segment of work into the setting, and the student begins to become disruptive, then you may need to move back a step, and further break down the task into more easily accomplished steps.

Criterion. Once Dave correctly points to the picture of assistance approximately 3–5 times in a row without teacher prompts and after completing a minimal amount of work, introduce new teachers and settings, where appropriate, followed by the introduction of new communicative responses (pictures).

The previous examples illustrated our attempts to teach individuals (who have been assessed to engage in behavior problems maintained by escape) to request assistance or escape from unpleasant situations. We will now turn to teaching attention-getting responses for those students who appear to exhibit problem behavior for social attention. *Readers should note that many of the general principles outlined in this section on escape are common to other training efforts.* For example, the emphasis on efficient prompt fading efforts is a consideration whether the goal is teaching assistance/escape response, requests for attention, requests for tangibles, or requests for sensory activities. Similarly, the focus on establishing "errorless" and appropriate environments for teaching as well as ensuring that the response being taught will be responded to as hoped, are important for all teaching efforts.

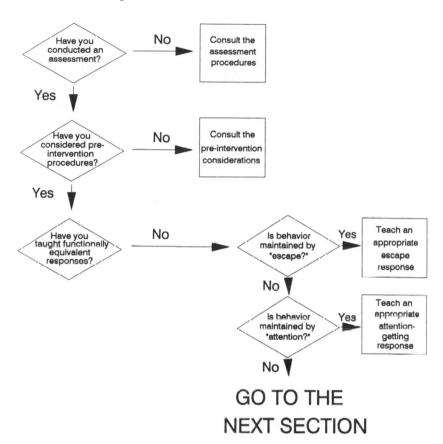

GO TO THE
NEXT SECTION

Teaching Requests for Attention

Teaching individuals how to request attention from others appropriately can be a difficult task. Aside from training this request so that it is elicited spontaneously, a critical concern expressed by many caregivers is the fear that the person will just substitute one annoying attention-getting response (e.g., screaming) with another (e.g., nagging the teacher). An individual who is constantly demanding the attention of others with signs or through verbal means can be as disruptive as someone who is acting aggressively or is engaging in tantrums. To illustrate just how disruptive some attention-getting behavior problems can be, we will describe some assessments conducted with a young woman who exhibited frequent self-injurious behavior.

Kate

Kate was 16 years old at the time of our assessment, and was living in a local developmental center. She displayed no verbal or signed speech and made her needs known through gestures. She was diagnosed as having autism and severe mental retardation. Kate's self-injurious behaviors included head banging and hand biting, and seemed to occur most frequently when she was left alone for even short periods of time. This observation was supported by results of administrations of the MAS to her teachers. Both teachers rated her self-injury as being maintained by social attention.

Interactions between Kate and her teachers were videotaped over a 2-month period. In observing these tapes, two patterns became quite apparent. First, the number of requests to perform tasks directed at Kate was quite high. Additionally, Kate's teachers spent an inordinate amount of time next to her. Kate was rarely left alone, and her teachers had for some time included her in most of their activities. Unfortunately, she would not complete work independently, and she was frequently a problem in group settings unless she was the focus of the group's attention. Kate's teachers complained that her progress was limited because of her requiring individual attention, and that she could not be easily handled without it. They felt drained working with her, and believed that the other students' progress was suffering because of their attention to Kate.

It is clear that this constant demand for attention can be a disruptive influence at home, at school, or at work. What is also clear is that Kate successfully manipulated the behavior of her teachers. They learned that if they spent a great deal of time with Kate she would be well behaved. The teachers were punished for leaving her alone by Kate's self-injury, which increased dramatically in these situations. If you look at Kate's self-injurious behavior as a form of nonverbal communication (i.e., communicating, "I want attention"), it is obvious that she is using it successfully.

Selecting the Training Setting

As mentioned in the chapter on "Preintervention Considerations," *the setting selected for teaching attention-getting responses is particularly critical for promoting successful generalization*. It is important *not* to rely too heavily on training in traditional one-to-one situations. Ideally, training should proceed in the setting where the student is likely to want to request attention. For example, teaching sessions can be carried out while the student is engaging in independent seat work, while engaging in other group activities, or after dinner in the living room while everyone is watching television. One way to determine the correct setting is to look at those times when the individual is engaging in most of their behavior problems. The scatter plot assessment described in Chapter 3 is a good formal method of conducting this analysis (Touchette et al., 1985).

High rates of attention-getting problem behavior in an after-lunch group setting, for example, would indicate that this might be a good place to teach a request for attention. In such a setting, it may be set up so that the student is participating in a group activity, and the teacher is sitting nearby, but out of direct view of the student. When the student is not the focus of attention from the group for a short period of time, the teacher could prompt a response from the student that might get the group leader's attention. This type of training arrangement is in contrast with the common practice of teaching in a one-to-one setting, and then hoping for generalization to groups. Recent work with one young woman illustrates how such training occurred at a job site.

LYDIA

Lydia was 25 years old at the time of assessment and was living in a group home. She had received various diagnoses, including Mild Mental Retardation and Dysthymia (characterized by depression). Her verbal communication skills were extensive, and she had some ability to describe how she felt about others. Lydia had been described as having a "low frustration tolerance," and did not get along well with peers.

This last description was a source of confusion for those who worked with Lydia because on one hand she seemed very interested in peers, yet she said she did not like the people with whom she worked and her interactions with them consisted mostly of arguments. It was this type of peer interaction problem that had resulted in her losing several jobs, and being asked to leave two previous group homes.

The MAS and records kept by the workshop staff indicated that these arguments may have been attempts to obtain peer attention. One interpretation was that because she lacked appropriate peer interaction skills, her only way of sustaining any prolonged interchange was to argue with others. It was decided that the target for Lydia was to teach her a variety of appropriate social interaction skills at the job site in order to give her another way to obtain peer attention.

This training took place at the workshop. Some initial role playing took place whereby Lydia was shown how to have a brief but pleasant conversation with a peer. Then, while she was working as part of an assembly line crew, the trainer would stand a few yards away and gesture for her to initiate a conversation. After about 60 seconds, she was prompted to end the conversation by saying, "Got to get back to work!". Prompting the end of the conversation was planned so that (1) she would not spend too much time away from her job, and (2) she would have less time to begin an argument. Within a few weeks the trainer faded out her involvement and allowed Lydia to initiate and terminate conversations herself. This intervention resulted in significant reductions in her arguments with peers at work.

In a variety of ways, Lydia was not typical of participants in our work. She clearly had many more skills than most of the persons with whom we have conducted functional communication training. However, the basic assumptions made about her behavior problems (i.e., that they were functional for her) seemed to be consistent with the findings of others with whom we have worked, despite her being included in a class of persons now considered to be "dually diagnosed."

Because of Lydia's rather extensive base of skills, communication training with her involved a more elaborate repertoire than we have taught to many of our other students (e.g., complex conversation skills versus asking for one or two objects in the environment). For this type of intervention, we have relied on the excellent work of others to assist us in these complex training procedures. We have adapted work with students labeled as juvenile delinquents (e.g., Goldstein & Glick, 1987), as well as with students with developmental disabilities (e.g., Gaylord–Ross, Haring, Breen, & Pitts–Conway, 1984; Hunt et al., 1985) in order to teach our students age-appropriate social and conversational skills. However, despite the inclusion of more elaborate skills training in this kind of work, this intervention differs from previous efforts by other investigators because of our consideration of the function of the behavior problem (e.g., to gain peer attention) in selecting the particular social skill to teach (e.g., a conversation which prolongs social interactions with peers; for an exception, see Hunt et al., 1988). In other words, we do not just teach social skills, but instead, attempt to select and teach those skills that will most likely provide the student with the types of consequences being elicited by his or her problem behavior.

Students with Good Communication Skills

Lydia's case points out an issue that is occasionally brought up when dealing with students who have good language skills. The typical question posed is, *"My student communicates quite well, but continues to engage in behavior problems. Why is that, and can I still use this approach?"* The usual response to this type of question is a series of additional questions about the student and the behavior: "Do you know why the student is disruptive?" "Have you conducted an assessment?" "Is the student spontaneously requesting things functionally related to the challenging behavior (e.g., attention, assistance, foods)?" "Are others providing these things when they are requested?" "Is the student making these requests at appropriate times?"

Although many individuals can satisfactorily answer most of these questions, it is the last one that is usually problematic. There are many students who can communicate. There are also students who can spontaneously ask for things they want, and those around them will usually provide these things when they are requested. The real question becomes, *do students always know what they want and when they want it*? It is important to note here that persons *without* severe handicaps often have difficulty identifying what it is they really want. For example, how many times have you felt sad, yet you did not know *why* you were sad? Did you ever find yourself getting angry at someone without really knowing why? Those readers with young children will quickly recognize this phenomenon. For example, it is not uncommon for a 2-year-old to ask for something, become upset when it is provided, ask for a second item instead, become upset when that is provided, and proceed to follow this pattern for a seemingly endless period of time. Although the child can say the right words, and has been successful in the past in getting things, we describe this as "not knowing what you want."

When discussing this issue with persons who do not have severe handicaps, therapists also refer to this as "lacking insight" or "not being in touch with your feelings." As evidenced by the number of psychologists and counselors currently employed in this country, it is clear that many of us have difficulty identifying want we want. And, clearly, much has been written (both pro and con) about the meaning and value of insight in improving people's lives (e.g., Barrett, Hampe, & Miller, 1978; Casey & Berman, 1985; Hartmann, Roper, & Gelfand, 1977). Relevant to the present discussion, however, is the fact that some of the students engaging in severe behavior problems may know *what* to say, but may not know *when* to say it.

Functional communication training for students who are good at communicating becomes less an issue of teaching specific communication skills, and more a job of teaching the student when to use the skills they already possess. It is interesting to note that the effect of gaining insight on one's problems has been described in ways that are not unlike the goals of functional communication training.

> Insight ... enable(s) the person to understand more clearly what he wants and how to go about getting it, by broadening the range of alternative ways of dealing with life situations that may be considered, and by fostering better discriminations between what is safe and what is unsafe to do ... (Wachtel, 1977; p. 93)

In Lydia's case, she already had an extensive verbal repertoire. Many times she would explain her outbursts as being due to her anger at others because of perceived slights made to her, and because of this she did not like to be around peers. However, the assessment indicated that despite the content of what she said (i.e., "I don't want to talk to them"), she really was acting in ways that would get her more peer attention rather than less.

The focus of intervention became teaching her to engage in ways that would appropriately gain attention from peers in those situations where she appeared to be most problematic. However, unlike many therapy situations (e.g., Alexander & French, 1946), no attempt was made to get her to verbalize that she really wanted to interact with peers. Instead, she was encouraged to act in ways that would gain her more enjoyable peer attention (i.e., pleasant conversations), an outcome that the assessment suggested she really wanted. By teaching her these skills, her disruptive behavior was all but eliminated within a few weeks, and peers reported her as being more pleasant to work with.

Selecting a response that will get the person access to appropriate attention can at times be difficult. As mentioned in the introduction to this section, the response itself should not be annoying to others. In the next example, work with a young woman who had very limited communication abilities is described. This example was selected in part because of the use of a response to provide assistance to get her access to adult attention.

VAL

Val was 21 years old at the time of our first contact. She was living in a group home with five other individuals, and attended a prevocational workshop program in a segregated school during the day. Val was well liked by those who worked with her, and she enjoyed the company of others. She had a variety of diagnoses, including Severe Mental Retardation and Congenital Rubella Syndrome. She also displayed profound visual and hearing deficits and could use only a few signs to communicate (e.g., bathroom, drink).

Val was referred because of the frequent outbursts she demonstrated. These episodes included screaming, slapping others and head butting, throwing any objects that were within her reach, and taking off her clothes. Data collected over a period of several months along with administrations of the MAS both in the group home and at the workshop revealed highly reliable reports that these behavior problems were most likely maintained by adult attention. It appeared that she would engage in tantrums if she were left alone for more than 5–10 minutes.

It was suggested that staff teach Val to sign "Help?" which would mean "May I help you?" This was chosen as an *attention-getting response* because it was to be followed by the staff members letting her accompany them while they were engaging in domestic tasks. Normally, staff members would prepare all meals, set and clear the table, and do the laundry on their own. This was also a time where Val was disruptive, apparently because the staff members were occupied with other activities and she had to sit alone for extended periods of time. Having Val request to help them with these tasks was seen as a good way to (1) provide her with adult attention, (2) have her begin to learn domestic routines, and (3) occupy her time during normally unscheduled times.

The staff had two main objections to this approach. First, *because she wasn't able to complete these tasks, they were concerned that she would become frustrated.* However, by having her participate at least partially in each task so that she could successfully complete a portion of the job, it was assumed that this would not be a problem (Baumgart, Brown et al., 1982; Baumgart, Vincent et al., 1982). Second, *there was a concern that, because she was disruptive so often during the day, now she would be constantly signing "Help?" and the staff would have to provide her with one-to-one attention throughout the day.* It was recommended that they attempt the training and assess just how often she was requesting attention.

Teaching Val to request attention by using the sign "Help?" was accomplished in a manner similar to previous descriptions of functional communication training. She was led to a chair in the living room, and was left alone for approximately 30 seconds. This duration was selected because it was a period of time the staff thought that she could sit by herself without being disruptive. After this delay, staff members physically prompted her to make the sign for "Help?" and then had her accompany them on some short errand (e.g., clearing the lunch dishes).

After the task was completed, she was again taken to a chair in the living room, and the teaching process just described was repeated. The prompts for her sign were faded, as described in Table 5-3. Delayed prompting and rapid fading of the physical guidance was used to get Val to sign "Help?" when she was sitting alone, without additional prompts.

Val progressed rapidly through these teaching steps, and appeared to enjoy the whole process. Within 3 weeks she was regularly signing "Help?" without teacher prompts, and the rate of her disruptive behavior declined significantly. In the first few weeks after she was successful in signing on her own, she began using the sign almost constantly. The staff members were encouraged to respond to *all* requests, and continue to monitor their frequency. *Within 2 weeks, the rate of her requests declined without further intervention to within a level that was acceptable to staff.* No subsequent increase in her disruptive behavior was observed.

This example points out that the observable content of a phrase or other form of communication is not as important as the effect it produces on others. In the present case, teaching Val to say "Help?" could be viewed as a means of showing her how to offer assistance. However, because it would reliably

TABLE 5-3. Prompt fading steps for teaching requests for attention

Phase	Prompt Level 1	Prompt Level 2	Prompt Level 3	Prompt Level 4	Student Response	Trainer Response
I	Student is sitting alone	Touches student's hand	Partial physical guidance to prompt sign	Full physical guidance to prompt sign	Students signs "Help?"	Accompanies student on domestic chore
II	Student is sitting alone	Touches student's hand	Partial physical guidance to prompt sign		Students signs "Help?"	Accompanies student on domestic chore
III	Student is sitting alone	Touches student's hand			Students signs "Help?"	Accompanies student on domestic chore
IV	Student is sitting alone				Students signs "Help?"	Accompanies student on domestic chore

elicit sustained attention from the staff, it was designed as an attention-getting response. And in this case, it was a response that elicited attention from the staff in a way that was not annoying—an important consideration in many settings.

An additional consideration illustrated here was initial staff resistance to include Val in domestic routines. This is an all-too-common occurrence in many residential placements. Typically, when the consumer or student leaves his or her residence for work or school, staff members use the time to make beds, do laundry, vacuum, and so on. It is also ironic that often the day placement is working on teaching these very same skills. The desire for efficiency in these situations can sometimes obscure an important opportunity to provide skills training. In the current example, *by allowing Val to participate partially in these chores, they not only provided her with appropriate attention, they also initiated the teaching of skills necessary for her future independence* (Baumgart, Brown, et al., 1982).

In the next section, we will turn our attention to teaching requests for tangibles. Again, all of the training considerations mentioned previously in the section on "Teaching Requests for Assistance/Escape" and in this section on "Teaching Requests for Attention" are applicable when teaching other communicative responses.

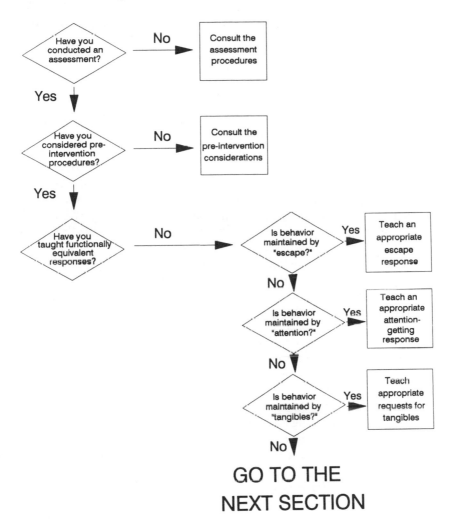

GO TO THE
NEXT SECTION

Teaching Requests for Tangibles

There are times when the results of assessments indicate that challenging behavior may not occur to escape difficult or boring tasks or to elicit attention from others. Rather, many of the individuals with whom we have worked appear to expend an inordinate amount of effort trying to get *things*. Instead of, or in addition to, wanting attention from others or escape from unpleasant situations, some persons with severe disabilities seem to display problem behavior in order to get such things as toys, foods, activities, or even certain privileges. One student with whom we worked illustrated this pattern quite clearly.

Robert

Robert was 18 years old at the time of initial referral. He was very large, weighing over 250 pounds, and would intimidate the staff with his outbursts. He could say a few words, which usually involved requests for food or his favorite magazine (a particular issue of *Sports Illustrated*). The extent of his ability to intimidate the staff was made clear just before a recent trip.

As students from Robert's residence were getting into a bus to go to a theme park, it was observed that in addition to a checklist that included the student's names, there was a place for "Robert's Magazine" on the checkoff sheet. When asked about this, staffers recalled a trip not too long ago when they inadvertently forgot to bring the magazine with them on the bus.

Approximately a half hour into a trip to a nearby zoo, Robert began saying "Magazine." The staff knew immediately that he wanted his favorite sports magazine, and to their horror realized that no one had remembered to bring it. Within a few seconds, Robert's face became red, his hands were clenched in a fist, and staff members knew it was only a matter of time before he would begin to strike out at anyone nearby. They quickly moved the others away from him, turned the bus around, and raced home to pick up the magazine.

In this case, no demands were being placed on Robert. There were a number of activities going on in the bus that presumably could have kept his interest. In addition, there was no lack of both staff and peer attention. What appeared to be eliciting his aggressive outbursts was the absence of this one object (his magazine). And, as was usually the case, the staff dealt with these episodes of aggression by giving him the magazine. Robert appeared to have learned that you first verbally request the magazine. However, if it is not forthcoming, a good way to ensure that he get the magazine was to be violently disruptive (sort of like saying, "Perhaps you didn't hear me, but I really want my magazine!").

When beginning functional communication training for students with challenging behavior presumably maintained by its tangible consequences, a number of interesting problems can arise. Typically, parents, teachers, and staff members ask questions such as "But, if you teach him how to ask for things, won't he ask for them too often?" "What if she asks for things I can't give her right now?" and "What if she asks for something I don't want to give her?" In addition, a more general question is often posed, "Isn't that just giving in to him?" Work with a young man named Randy highlights many of these issues.

Randy

Randy was 23 years old and lived in a group home in a major metropolitan city. His communication skills were severely limited, and usually involved some gestures. He was liked by both the staff at his group home, and at a local day placement where he worked on contracts obtained by the agency (e.g., putting parts into plastic bags). He had been diagnosed as having severe mental retardation.

Several times a day, Randy would throw his work material off his table, scream loudly, and fall on the floor. This was of concern, not only because of the missed work, and the limitations it placed on him for alternate employment, but also because he would sometimes injure others by hitting them with the work materials.

During discussions with staff following preliminary assessments, one person pointed out that much of this disruptive behavior seemed to center around coffee. One interpretation was that when he wanted coffee but couldn't get it, he would scream and thrash about on the floor. When other staff members were questioned about this, they indicated that he did receive coffee throughout the day in the form of task consequences. If he performed a predetermined amount of work, they would give him a small drink of coffee. Yet, he was still being disruptive, presumably to get more coffee.

Based on this information, it was suggested that he be allowed to request coffee whenever he wanted by pointing to his empty coffee cup. More sophisticated forms of communication were ruled out, based on previous unsuccessful efforts at teaching him verbal and sign language. Many of the staffers were unhappy with this intervention suggestion. They expressed a variety of concerns, including whether he would become unmotivated to work if coffee was given to him "free," whether he would request coffee constantly and receive too much during the day, and whether or not this constituted "giving in" to him.

Partly as a result of these concerns, it was recommended that data be collected on task performance and amount of coffee consumed both pre- and postintervention to evaluate the effects of teaching him to request coffee. Staff were told that this would be a temporary experiment, and that we would evaluate the positive and negative effects of the program after several weeks.

Teaching Randy to communicate this request was relatively easy. Pointing to the empty coffee cup was selected because he already had a response that approximated this effort, and it could be recognized as a request for coffee from almost anyone in the program. After a short period of time during which he was required to work on a task, he was physically and verbally prompted to point to the cup in the presence of the coffee pot. In the past, his seeing the coffee pot appeared to be a signal for disruptive behavior, and it was hoped that it could be used instead to signal the request for coffee. Table 5-4 illustrates the prompt fading steps used with Randy.

Initially, the coffee pot was visible during training because its presence often signaled the onset of his screaming. It was assumed that the coffee pot was a reminder for him to get coffee. Ultimately, however, the coffee pot was placed out of sight. This was done to get him to request coffee even if someone forgot to get the pot.

Within a few days, Randy was reliably pointing to the empty coffee cup, and was receiving coffee each time he did this. After 3 weeks it was observed that, (1) the frequency of his disruptive behavior was reduced to near-zero levels, (2) he was spontaneously pointing to the empty cup of coffee, (3) task performance was maintained at preintervention levels even though he could have constant access to the reinforcer, and (4) his preintervention level of coffee drinking was approximately four cups of coffee per day, and the postintervention level of drinking was approximately five cups per day (decaffeinated). The intervention appeared successful, without seeing excessive requests for coffee, and without decrements in task performance.

But Won't They Ask for It Too Often?

As mentioned above, parents, teachers, and other caregivers often express concern that if they teach an appropriate request for some favorite food, object, or activity, the student will use it so frequently that it too will become disruptive. In fact, this concern is frequently articulated regardless of the type of response being taught. Whether it is a request for food or drink as in Randy's case, a request for time away from work being taught to a student with escape-maintained behavior problems, or a request for social attention being taught to a person with behavior problems maintained by its social consequences, *there is a fear that the student will spend his or her day making requests at the expense of all other activities.*

Fortunately, *results from research using functional communication training indicate that students do not usually "abuse" their use of requests* (Bird et al., 1989; Durand & Carr, in press). It is often the case that initially the student will use the new skill to request tangibles (or any other goal) a great deal of the time; but within a few weeks these high frequency requests stabilize at an acceptable level. This decline in requests is frequently observed even without specific fading procedures.

Why don't participants request these reinforcers at higher rates? One explanation for this observation is *satiation*. In other words, once the student has constant access to food, social attention, a break from work, or any other reinforcer, the value of these stimuli to the student declines. To use an analogy, someone who is dieting may spend a great deal of time thinking

TABLE 5-4. Prompt fading steps for teaching requests for tangibles

Phase	Prompt Level 1	Prompt Level 2	Prompt Level 3	Prompt Level 4	Student Response	Trainer Response
I	Student is sitting alone with coffee pot out of sight	Student is sitting alone with coffee pot in sight	Partial physical guidance to prompt gesture	Full physical guidance to prompt gesture	Student points to empty coffee cup	Puts coffee in student's cup
II	Student is sitting alone with coffee pot out of sight	Student is sitting alone with coffee pot in sight	Partial physical guidance to prompt gesture		Student points to empty coffee cup	Puts coffee in student's cup
III	Student is sitting alone with coffee pot out of sight	Student is sitting alone with coffee pot in sight			Student points to empty coffee cup	Puts coffee in student's cup
IV	Student is sitting alone with coffee pot out of sight				Student points to empty coffee cup	Puts coffee in student's cup

and talking about food. A drive past an ice cream store may be torture because the dieter can't go in and have ice cream. However, if the same person stops dieting and eats whatever they choose, then the sight of something like ice cream no longer seems that important. Having constant access to food, attention, breaks from work, and so on, should make these stimuli less important.

In a similar manner, the relative *efficiency* of the new communicative response could also account for its less frequent use. For example, a student may spend most of the day engaging in self-injurious behavior to get some favorite snack (e.g., potato chips). And, this disruptive behavior may occasionally be successful in obtaining the food (e.g., maybe once in about every 20 episodes—or 5% of the time). If the student can request this snack and gain access to it at any time (i.e., 100% of the time), then you would expect that even though he or she appeared to be constantly "asking" for potato chips with self-injury, these new "requests" would have to occur far less often to get the same amount or even more chips. If the student had to be disruptive 20 times to get potato chips, and now only has to ask for it once, you should see requests occurring approximately 20 times less often than the self-injury. Presumably because of both satiation and response efficiency, concerns about the excessive use of the new communicative responses are often unfounded.

It is essential that the requests made by the students be responded to each time they are made, especially in the initial stages of teaching. Unless the student learns that this new response will be more successful in obtaining preferred reinforcers than using problem behavior, no reductions in the behavior problems will be observed. In a recent visit to a program that was attempting to use functional communication training with one student, this issue was highlighted. Staff members had given the student tokens on which were written the word "soda." They assessed that his dangerous aggressive behaviors were partially maintained by tangible consequences, and they were trying to get him to communicate appropriately for his favorite reinforcer—soda. Unfortunately, however, they reported that this intervention was not successful in reducing his aggression, and they were attempting to get permission to use contingent electric shock as a means of eliminating this behavior. A brief observation of the communication program in action revealed what may have been the problem with the intervention. On one occasion the student handed a staff member the token for soda, and the staff responded by saying "Not now, you have to wait until 3 P.M." Clearly, *the program as it was being carried out violated the main premise of functional communication training—the student requests something that is functionally related to his or her problem behavior and receives it.* If the request is not responded to reliably during the initial stages of training, it is expected that students will return to their previous means of obtaining things from the environment—through challenging behavior.

Teaching Delay of Gratification

Obviously, there are times when a student either must wait for the requested object or activity, or cannot have access to it at all. Before discussing either of these situations, it needs to be pointed out that readers should take care to ensure that the delay or refusal to provide some reinforcer is based on reasonable educational/clinical decisions. As mentioned in the Assessment chapter, there are times when parents, teachers, and/or staff members make decisions based on their own convenience, rather than on what is best for the student. Issues of convenience need to be balanced with the needs of the student.

Asking for a mother's attention when she is on the phone, requesting help from a teacher when he or she is working with another student, or seeking permission to go swimming on a day when no transportation is available are all examples of appropriate requests that may not be responded to immediately. Recall that initial training for functional communication training involves providing the requested object or activity following the request. Training is set up such that (1) the request can be provided, and (2) someone is always available during training to respond. Experience suggests that within a few weeks after successful intervention, students begin to tolerate delays such as those described above fairly well. Because of this, it is recommended that the staff wait to build in or test delays until after the program has been successful for at least 2 weeks.

In those cases where the ability of the student to wait for a response continues to be unacceptable, specific training procedures such as "Red Light Green Light" have been implemented after the initial success of communication training. This type of delay training has been used with students who may not be able to understand basic concepts of time (e.g., "You can watch TV at 6:30"). Training occurs with a green card on the student's table, which signals that all requests will be responded to immediately. For brief periods of time (several seconds to several minutes), a red card is placed on the table, and this signals that communicative responses will not be answered. During this brief time, all appropriate requests are ignored. Training proceeds slowly and gradually until delays that approximate those the student is likely to encounter are reached with little or no disruption.

Requests that Can't Be Fulfilled

When a student appears to want something that may never be available (e.g., visits with a family that no longer desires contact, eating inedibles, playing with fire, running out into the street), attempts are made to provide equivalent consequences in a form that can be provided. For example, although a student may appear to get upset in order to run outside and into the street, letting the student request running into the street would obviously not be appropriate. An analysis of the function of this behavior may indicate that running outside serves both to gain attention from teachers (who must run out after the student), and to escape from academic tasks. Therefore, the student would be taught to communicate for attention and escape (perhaps taking a break from work that would include time with the teacher). We attempt to find alternative means of approximating what the student appears to be requesting.

Using another example, a teacher complained recently that her student appeared to want to choose from among a variety of tasks instead of having the same task presented at the same time each day. The concern was that in regular classrooms, students are somewhat structured in that they have to take a math class at say 9:30, reading at 10:30, and so on. It was suggested that although math may have to be taught between 9:30 and 10:30, the student could still be provided with choices of math work. In other words, the student could be allowed to choose from among several types of problems to work on first, then second, etc. Being creative, parents, teachers, and staff should always be able to find opportunities to provide at least part of what the student wants.

Anticipating Student Requests/Frequent Prompting

An issue that we frequently confront in functional communication training is the use of too many prompts. *Parents, teachers, and staff members often spend a great deal of time anticipating what their students want.* In fact, many are very good at picking up subtle cues from their students as to what they want at any particular time. This behavior is reinforced because it can result in avoiding many problems. For example, suppose a student does not spontaneously communicate the need to go to the bathroom. If a teacher can anticipate this need by taking the student to the bathroom before an accident, cleaning up a mess is avoided, along with a possible tantrum. In the course of these activities, however, the teacher can inadvertently discourage student initiations of certain requests. Not waiting until the student makes a request can encourage what has been referred to as "prompt dependence," an overreliance on trainer prompts. The following case exemplifies the problems one can expect with *too much* anticipation.

PAUL

Paul was a 14-year-old student with autism who engaged in frequent aggression and self-injury. He had a long history of displaying these behaviors, and was making little progress in his academic program because of them. An assessment indicated that one important influence on his challenging behavior was the tangible consequences which frequently followed these responses. Following this assessment, it was suggested that he be taught to communicate requests for favorite tangibles.

We began functional communication training by teaching him to point to favorite objects and activities depicted as pictures on index cards. In the beginning of training, Paul's teacher would present the cards and wait for him to point to one of the objects. The teacher was instructed to give him what he pointed to. However, there were many times when Paul didn't seem to want what he pointed to and the teacher would then prompt him by saying "Do you want this (another choice)?" The teacher would then continue to prompt until he gave some sign that she had picked something he wanted. More and more, Paul began not to pay attention to the cards, but appeared to wait until the teacher happened to say the name of the object he wanted at that time. Paul rarely initiated requests through the use of the cards, but waited until his teacher prompted his responses. No reduction in his aggression or self-injury were observed during the program.

The strategy used by Paul's teacher involved reading nonverbal cues (e.g., his moving away, frowning) to suggest that Paul may not have wanted the object he pointed to. What is wrong with this strategy? First, for some students, these nonverbal cues may not be an accurate means of assessing their desires. For example, just because a student may frown when you say the phrase "Do you want to play with your truck?" may not mean that the student wouldn't enjoy playing with the truck if it was presented.

More importantly, however, by giving the student reinforcers without first expecting a response, the student may stop responding spontaneously. In Paul's case, he found that the easiest thing to do was to wait until the teacher mentioned some preferred activity. This was more efficient than (a) scanning all of the pictures, (b) matching a picture to a desired activity, and (c) pointing to the picture of interest. Perhaps because he sometimes made mistakes (i.e., he would inadvertently point to something he didn't like), Paul did not point to the pictures on his own. In fact, it took approximately 6 months of periodic feedback to Paul's teacher to get her to fade out the prompts. This fading of the prompts ultimately resulted in his using the pictures spontaneously, and reduced the frequency of his aggression and self-injury.

In the next section we discuss intervention suggestions for behaviors maintained by their sensory consequences. Although these behaviors can be viewed as distinct from socially mediated behavior problems (such as behaviors maintained by adult attention), readers should notice the heuristic value in adopting a communication model.

Teaching Requests for Alternate Sensory Activities

Behavior that is maintained by its sensory consequences can be most difficult to change. For behaviors controlled by their social consequences,

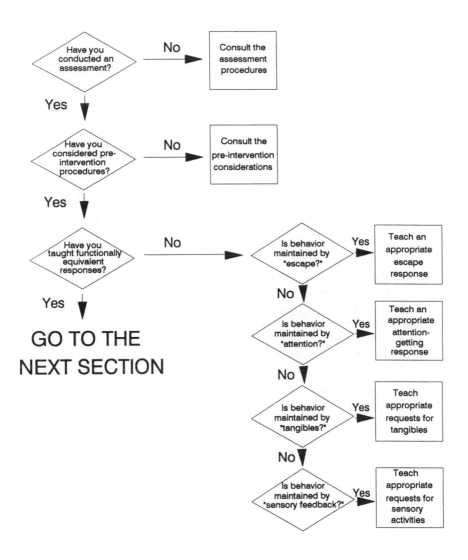

we can change various aspects of the social environment as a means of intervention. We can ignore attention-maintained behavior. We can "work through" (i.e., continue to present demands) those behaviors maintained by escape. And, we can withhold tangibles for behavior maintained by tangible consequences. Unfortunately, however, it is often difficult if not impossible to remove the consequences provided by sensory-maintained behavior. Our experience suggests that although these behaviors tend to be less severe in their intensity when compared to some behaviors maintained by social stimuli, intervention for behavior maintained by nonsocial stimuli is frequently more problematic. Again, this may be due to the inability to manipulate easily the variables maintaining these behaviors (e.g., sensory feedback).

It was mentioned in the Introduction that this aspect of functional communication training has received very little systematic attention. To date, we have not conducted controlled investigations on behavior maintained by sensory consequences that are comparable to the studies carried out with socially mediated behavior. Yet, because we have implemented interventions in this area, our preliminary efforts are reported here. *It is important to repeat, however, that this work goes beyond our data, and readers should be especially cautious in implementing these procedures.*

When discussing functional communication training in the context of behavior maintained by sensory feedback, using the communication model or metaphor we have adopted up to this point may be less obvious. One can look at behavior that, for example, serves to obtain adult attention as a form of communication because of the social nature of the response. This type of interaction (i.e., requesting attention) is consistent with generally held views of communication. On the other hand, it is more difficult to conceptualize behavior that is self-reinforcing as communicative. Despite this apparent problem, it appears useful to extend a communication model to sensory-maintained behavior for purposes of assessment and intervention design.

Following the logic outlined in previous sections, *assessment involves an analysis of the variables maintaining these behaviors (e.g., tactile input), and intervention includes both changes in the environment (e.g., efforts to "enrich" the current setting) and the teaching of a functionally equivalent behavior (e.g., an appropriate behavior that provides tactile stimulation).* And, because participants who engage in frequent sensory-maintained behaviors often lack meaningful social-communicative repertoires, teaching a social request for access to the sensory activity is usually included (e.g., a request such as "May I use the exercise bicycle?"). Work with Dale will illustrate this process.

Dale

Dale was a 23-year-old man who lived in a group home with seven other adults. Dale had limited social-communicative skills, and the group home staff frequently had difficulty anticipating his needs. He could perform most daily living skills with prompting, and appeared to enjoy being by himself.

Dale attended a community vocational program 5 days per week, and it was here that the staff reported frequent behavior problems. Most noticeable of these was Dale's frequent, and sometimes violent, rocking. If he was not currently engaged in an activity, he would begin to rock back and forth in a stereotyped manner. Occasionally he would rock so violently that he would knock over his rather large and heavy worktable, causing concern for his safety as well as for those around him.

Using the scatter plot described in the Assessment chapter, the staff found that the rocking was most frequent during "down times." This was especially true if there were periods during the day with more than 15 minutes without an activity. Administration of the MAS suggested that Dale's rocking may have been maintained by its sensory consequences.

With the findings from both the scatter plot and the MAS, several recommendations were made. First, it was suggested that the staff attempt to reduce the amount of time Dale spent without an activity. There appeared to be two or three times each day when he was unoccupied for more than 30 minutes. The program staff members were sympathetic to this suggestion, but explained that because of staff shortages, and because Dale was not yet working independently, they were not able to provide him with constant supervision.

In discussing this staffing problem, it was observed that there was one other participant in this program who, like Dale, required moderately high levels of prompting to continue working. *The suggestion was made that they explicitly target working with minimal supervision for these two adults because of the problems that arose when they were not supervised and because of the importance of working for periods of time without prompts.* It was recommended that they have these two adults work in a group with two adults who required less supervision. Using a combination of delayed and unpredictable feedback with this group, it was expected that "down time" could be reduced (see Dunlap & Johnson, 1985; Dunlap, Koegel, Johnson, & O'Neill, 1987; Dunlap, Plienis, & Williams, 1987).

The second recommendation involved selecting an alternate sensory activity to replace Dale's rocking. This activity should be age-appropriate and not interfere with community acceptance. It was suggested that riding an exercise bicycle might be an appropriate alternative that could provide him with sensory input comparable to his rocking. Unfortunately, previous attempts to encourage Dale to use the bike had been unsuccessful. To remedy this, the staff was instructed to have Dale sit on the bike several times per day and encourage him to peddle for a few seconds. If he seemed to enjoy the activity he could stay on the bike. If he did not appear to want to continue peddling they were to help him off the bike and back to work. Initially, Dale chose to get off the bike almost immediately. However, within a few weeks, the staff reported that he somehow learned to enjoy the peddling and that he had to be prompted to get off the bike after 5–10 minutes.

Once Dale had an appropriate alternate response (exercising on the bicycle), training focused on getting him to request the bike. It was decided to teach Dale to point to a picture of the exercise bike as a means of requesting this activity. Under the picture was written the phrase, "May I ride the bike?" so that staff members unfamiliar with the program could more easily understand the request. The prompting and prompt fading steps outlined in Table 5-5 were followed for approximately 2 months until he would successfully point to the picture without prompts.

Following these two interventions (i.e., training to work with less supervision, and teaching him to request riding the bike), Dale's rocking decreased to acceptable levels. The violent rocking occurred only rarely (i.e., less than once per month versus several times per day prior to intervention), and normally he would calmly rock back and forth only on the bus or in his bedroom.

TABLE 5-5. Prompt fading steps for teaching requests for exercise bicycle

Phase	Prompt Level 1	Prompt Level 2	Prompt Level 3	Prompt Level 4	Student Response	Trainer Response
I	Student is sitting alone	Picture is presented	Partial physical guidance to point to picture	Full physical guidance to point to picture	Student points to picture of exercise bike	Lets student ride on exercise bike
II	Student is sitting alone	Picture is presented	Partial physical guidance to point to picture		Student points to picture of exercise bike	Lets student ride on exercise bike
III	Student is sitting alone	Picture is presented			Student points to picture of exercise bike	Lets student ride on exercise bike
IV	Student is sitting alone	Picture is available			Student points to picture of exercise bike	Lets student ride on exercise bike

Environmental Assessment and Intervention

Environmental assessment and intervention is perhaps most important for sensory-maintained behavior problems. If a learner engages in multiple and frequent "self-stimulatory" behaviors, then it suggests that the student is not receiving sufficient stimulation from the prevailing social and physical environment. This is most obvious with students with dually sensory impairments (deaf and blind) who, presumably because of the lack of input from the environment, often engage in frequent stereotyped behavior (sometimes called "blindisms"). Assessment of Dale's rocking also supported this hypothesis and indicated that he was rocking most frequently when he had nothing to do. An integral part of his intervention therefore involved providing him with more stimulation through work activities.

This issue is especially relevant in large "institutional" settings. For example, a staff member at a nursing home recently requested assistance for one older woman's self-injury. It appeared that there was a 3-hour block in the afternoon during which time residents in wheelchairs were placed in a large room with a television set. None of the residents in this group had formal communication skills, and it was during this "leisure time" that the woman in question would repeatedly hit her head in a stereotypical manner. Initial discussion suggested that this behavior was being maintained by its sensory consequences, and that a first intervention would be to provide activities during leisure time. Staff members indicated they were too busy during this time to interact with these residents, and that they were requesting some intervention that would not involve significant staff effort.

It was pointed out that this was not an acceptable situation, and that staffing priorities would need to change before any intervention suggestion would be made. Several recommendations were made for changing staffing patterns so that someone would be available to interact with the residents during this time (for example, see Durand, 1983; 1985). This case illustrates that there are certain times when staff, teachers, or parents may not be able to interact with our students. However, it is reasonable to expect a minimal level of supervision throughout the day.

As alluded to above, *the functional analysis should have implications for both the communicative response to be taught and for environmental modifications.* For example, if a student is engaging in problem behavior maintained by escape, then in addition to teaching the student to request breaks or assistance, staff should look to the environment to see just what the student wants to escape from. It may be that the tasks presented are too difficult or too boring. It also may be that the setting may be too noisy or crowded, and the student is attempting physically to escape. *It is important to view these behavior problems as indicating both a skills deficit on the part of the student, and a possible deficit on the part of the prevailing environment.* More discussion of environmental interventions is available from other sources (see, Meyer & Evans, 1989).

Reinforcer Sampling

Dale's case also illustrates another problem often encountered when attempting to select alternative sensory activities. Initially Dale didn't like the exercise bike. Yet, after being provided with several opportunities to sample this activity (also known as *reinforcer sampling;* Ayllon & Azrin, 1968; Holz, Azrin, & Ayllon, 1963; Sulzer–Azaroff & Mayer, 1977), he appeared to learn how to provide himself with the same type of sensory feedback previously obtained by rocking. It is important that attempts be made to introduce new activities to students. This may be particularly important because many of the activities enjoyed by students like Dale may not be age-appropriate (e.g., a 35-year-old man who constantly manipulates a rag doll) and may interfere with community acceptance. This issue is highlighted again in our work with Deryk.

DERYK

Deryk was a 26-year-old man who was referred to us because of his chronic "toe-picking." Deryk had adequate verbal skills and could carry on a limited conversation with others. Due to spina bifida Deryk's mobility was limited and, at the time of referral, he was using a wheelchair. He especially enjoyed social activities and writing.

Deryk's toe-picking involved the pulling off of skin from his toes, which invariably resulted in serious infections. Staff had a variety of explanations to explain his self-injury. Some hypothesized that he was deliberately injuring his toes in order to sabotage efforts to get him out of the wheelchair and using crutches. Others felt that the accompanying attention (i.e., reprimands to stop, medical attention to prevent infections) was maintaining this self-injury. Observations over several months and the use of the MAS suggested that picking at the skin around his toes may have been maintained by its sensory consequences.

Previous consultations with Deryk had also implied that the sensory feedback provided by toe picking was important in its continued occurrence. It had been suggested that in order to provide him with comparable feedback, he should be allowed to keep his feet in sand at home and at work. Although at the time this recommendation was acceptable to the staff, it quickly became clear that this was not a practical solution to the problem. Because of lack of portability, and because of the way it made him stand out among peers, and so forth, the suggestion was never fully carried out.

In order to address these issues, Deryk's reinforcer preferences were surveyed. It was found that he liked pens, which he used to doodle on paper, his favorite color was black, and that he took pride in his ownership of certain things. Based on this information, it was suggested that the staff help Deryk purchase a black pen and have his name engraved on it. In addition, he should be allowed to carry the pen with him to work and he should be encouraged to use the pen to doodle and to hold and manipulate it throughout the day. This suggestion incorporated both an age-appropriate sensory activity with several components of his favorite reinforcers. No conclusions from this recent intervention have yet been determined.

Deryk's case illustrates the need to find creative solutions to the unique problems often posed by our students. How do you get a student who appears to be highly motivated to pick at his skin to substitute it with some other activity that is not harmful, won't interfere with his progress, and will not serve to ostracize him in the community? Again, throughout this book we have attempted to provide guidelines that will need to be adapted for each student and each environment.

Multiple Motivations

As described both in the section on the conceptualization and in the Assessment chapter, for some individuals, behavior problems can be multiply motivated. A particular behavior can be used for various reasons in a variety of settings. For example, a student can use screaming at school to escape academic tasks, and use screaming at home to get parental attention. One solution to this situation is to teach the student different communicative responses in each setting to match the function of the behavior problem. For example, the student just described could be taught to ask for help at school, and could be taught to request parental attention appropriately at home. It is likely that students will need to be taught a variety of responses, depending on their needs and the requirements of each setting.

But what about students whose behaviors are multiply motivated in the same setting? What if they use their problem behavior simultaneously to get attention, escape from work, obtain tangibles, and so on? This is a frequently asked question, and one where there is little advice available that is data-based. Our approach has been first to assure that the assessment was carried out properly. This means checking that (1) the behavior problems were defined specifically enough, and (2) the settings in which the asssessments are conducted are also delimited properly. It has often been the case (as mentioned in the Assessment chapter) that improper grouping together of several behaviors has led to conclusions that behaviors are multiply motivated. Similarly, attempting to assess behavior problems in multiple settings (e.g., "at school") rather than in specific settings (e.g., "in one-to-one teaching settings") has also led to the assumption of multiple motivations.

However, there have been occasions where we felt that the assessment was adequate, and still two or more stimuli appeared to be controlling the behavior problem. An example is illustrated below.

Bernie

Bernie was 14 years old at the time he was referred to us. He was diagnosed as having Severe Mental Retardation and San Filippo Syndrome, a degenerative neurological condition. He engaged in delayed and immediate echolalia and perseverative speech, rarely using speech appropriately. Of concern to his parents and teachers was his self-injurious behaviors. He would bang his hand forcefully on tables, pull his hair, and bite his bottom lip.

Assessments including administrations of the MAS suggested that two influences may be controlling these behaviors. Both adult attention and escape from academic tasks seemed to be important in controlling these behavior problems. And, *the effects of attention and escape appeared to be exacerbated by two setting events: fatigue and hunger.* He seemed to require more attention and would tolerate tasks less when he was tired or hungry.

The intervention strategy for Bernie involved providing him with snacks during the day, attempting to intervene on his nighttime sleep problems, and trying to find a response that would simultaneously provide him with access to adult attention and provide him with an appropriate escape from work. It was felt that teaching him a response that would only accomplish one or the other would result in less than optimal results. He probably would not like a break from work, for example, if he had to take it alone. Similarly, he probably would not like additional attention from others as much if he had to continue working at the same time.

One solution was to teach him to ask to take things down to the principal's office. This was an activity he would engage in at various times during the day for the teacher, especially when the teacher thought he looked tired. This job got him away from the academic tasks briefly, and also allowed him to interact with the staff in the office. Because his verbal skills were limited, he was provided with a picture of the office to which he could point.

His teachers reported that he quickly learned to point to the picture to leave the classroom, and that his self-injury was significantly reduced. This success was attributed to the communication intervention because the implementation of the snacks and intervention for sleep problems occurred after the positive results were initially observed. And as we have often seen, Bernie's teachers were surprised to find that he continued to work in class, and appeared to enjoy the in-class work more than before intervention.

Again, this is one of just a few cases where we have determined multiple motivations for a particular behavior problem. Our solution was one that hopefully fit his needs as well as those of his teachers. It is obvious that further work is needed in this area to identify the extent to which behavior problems are multiply motivated, and intervention strategies to deal with them.

What follows next is a detailed discussion of how we respond to instances of problem behavior. Because these procedures are likely to be misunderstood with only a cursory study, it is hoped that readers will spend some time on the next section to understand the procedures and their rationales.

Response-Independent Consequences

Perhaps the first introduction persons in this area get to behavior problems involves training in how to deliver consequences. Almost all parent training, staff training, and teacher training programs allocate major portions of their time discussing the variety of consequences available for intervention. And, in the past, there were good reasons for this heavy emphasis. There is an extensive literature on the effects of procedures such as contingent time-out, overcorrection, reprimands, physical restraint, and contingent electric shock on the frequency of problem behavior (Carr & Lovaas, 1983; Foxx & Bechtel, 1983; Harris & Ersner–Hershfield, 1978). For some time, this approach to intervention was one of the few systematically documented intervention methods and appeared to be an easy solution to these disturbing problems.

Despite the emphasis traditionally placed on consequence-based interventions, there is a planned attempt to de-emphasize these specific procedures in this book. Readers should note that we have decided *not* to include an extensive review of the literature involving the use of such interventions, nor is there any discussion of how to implement these procedures (for reviews, see Durand & Carr, 1989; Favell et al., 1982; Foxx & Bechtel, 1983). Instead, given the model adopted by this approach (see Chapter 2), we take a different view of consequences.

If a student should engage in problem behavior, try not to intervene in any way.

The reason why we do not recommend intervention if a student "acts up" is because we want the student to begin to learn that misbehavior will no

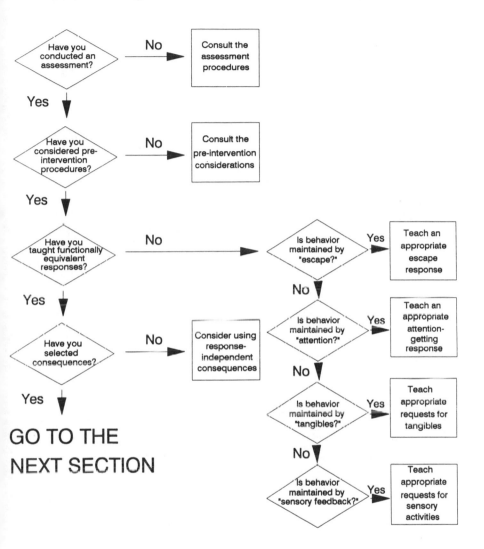

longer have an effect on the environment. Suppose, for example, that in general a student does not want to work on the tasks that are available. However, during one trial of training, as you are prompting him or her to the break area, the student becomes interested in the work materials and wants to continue working. Further suppose that as you prompt him or her to get up, the student hits you and starts screaming, and you now tell her to sit back down. Although your goal was not to reinforce the student with a break following the tantrum, you instead may have reinforced the student for the tantrum by allowing him or her to continue working. A real example of this problem was observed by us a number of years ago with a young man named Pete.

Pete

Pete was 14 years old at the time we met him, he had no formal communication system, and he was living on a "behavioral unit" in an institution. Pete was well liked by the staff, despite the fact that he often engaged in rather serious tantrums, which included head hitting on the floor. One program that he was involved with was a toileting plan. It appeared that he would have frequent toileting accidents, so it was decided to use overcorrection to attempt to eliminate this problem.

The overcorrection program involved having staff stand behind him, hold his hands on a mop, and make him slowly mop up the floor for 25 minutes after each toileting accident. This program was quite aversive for staff (in fact, there were reports that many staff would overlook accidents to avoid running the program), and appeared aversive to Pete. Despite the apparent aversiveness of this program, incidents of toileting accidents were increasing.

One possible reason for the increase in these accidents became obvious one day during change of shift. This was the time during the day (at about 3:30 P.M.) when staff members of the morning and evening shifts were in the nurses' station exchanging information. At one point during the meeting there was a loud bang on the plexiglass window coming from the far side of the station. Three or four staff members came running over to investigate, just in time to watch Pete pull down his pants and urinate on the floor. Pete was the person who banged on the window in an apparent effort to bring his "accident" to the attention of staff.

At first this puzzled staff. Why would anyone deliberately want to participate in such an aversive program? Theories of masochism abounded, until it was pointed out that perhaps the overcorrection program had become reinforcing. Maybe because Pete had no other way to gain staff attention, he learned that one reliable method was to urinate everywhere but in the bathroom. In fact, it was discovered that a large number of the accidents occurred during times when staff attention was least available (e.g., during change of shift). It appeared that he learned to use urination as a nonverbal means to communicate "I want attention," even though that attention came in the form of an overcorrection procedure.

This example illustrates the possible detrimental effects of trying to intervene when a student misbehaves. *Even a presumably aversive intervention can, depending on the context, serve to reinforce problem behavior.* What we advocate is not to change the ongoing interaction as a function of student misbehavior. Not only are we saying to avoid planned consequences, it is also recommended that you *continue your interaction with the student as before, even if you believe it might be reinforcing*. Therefore, if you are prompting a student to a break area when she becomes aggressive, continue to prompt him or her to take a break. Likewise, if you are directing the student back to work when he or she becomes disruptive, continue your efforts to get the student back to work. If you are praising a student and he or she screams, continue to praise. And, if you are offering a supposed favorite food (e.g., candy), and the student hits you, continue to offer the food. The message you want to communicate to the student is "your problem behavior no longer has an effect on us—however, if you use a behavior that is appropriate we will give you what you want."

A major reason why we intervene in this way is that we do not know why any particular student engages in any individual behavior at any specific point in time. As we saw in Chapter 2, the field has made progress in determining why a student might, in general, be engaging in certain behaviors under certain conditions. It may be possible, for example, to determine that screaming and hand hitting in group settings *probably* serves to get attention in many cases. However, at any one time, there is no way to know why a student just screamed or just bit his or her arm. Because it is difficult if not impossible to evaluate the variables controlling each instance of a behavior, we don't try. Instead, we try not to let any particular consequence follow the behavior (e.g., more attention or less attention).

Although this strategy seems to contradict traditional behavioral teaching approaches, we find it consistent with classic learning models of behavior. For example, researchers in the area of Pavlovian conditioning have used what is called a "truly random" control group to obtain a baseline on behavior (Prokasy, 1965; Rescorla, 1967). Prior to this work, researchers compared the effects of pairing of a CS (e.g., a light) and a UCS (e.g., a shock; i.e., the light means shock is coming), with a control condition in which the CS was never paired with the UCS (i.e., they never occur together). What Prokasy and Rescorla pointed out was that despite the intention that this control serve as a "no learning" condition, In fact this latter condition was a situation in which learning did occur. What is learned is that, in the present example, the light is a safety signal, and that the light signals a period of time when no shock is coming. In their truly random control, they set up a situation where the light and the shock were presented randomly. Sometimes the shock came on before the light, sometimes after, and sometimes concurrently. The message here is that the light and the shock are independent. When they are presented randomly, having the light on tells you nothing about the shock.

Similarly, work in operant psychology has introduced a procedure known as response-independent reinforcer delivery (Catania, 1984). Here, known reinforcers are presented randomly, sometimes at the same time as a particular response, and sometimes not. In a manner similar to the truly random control condition for classical conditioning, response-independent reinforcers are occasionally used in research with animals to assess the effects of terminating contingencies (Boakes, 1973; Rescorla & Skucy, 1969). Responding in a certain way results in no predictable reaction from the environment.

This is relevant for our work because what we are trying to accomplish are response-independent consequences for problem behavior. *The goal is to let the student know that behavior problems will not affect others in any predictable way.* It is important to note here that educators, parents, and professionals often relate to us that they are already doing this. They explain that their typical response to a behavior problem is to ignore it. But are they really not responding? An example will help illustrate when even "ignoring" can be a reinforcer.

Carol

Carol was a 6-year-old girl who had received a diagnosis of autism. Her language abilities were extremely limited, and she would rely upon vocalizations and pointing to obtain things that she wanted. Carol was referred to us because of the frequent and severe tantrums that she exhibited. She would often begin screaming, bite her hand, and thrash around on the floor when she became upset.

Carol's teachers and her parents would respond to these tantrums by "ignoring" them. If she became upset, they would remove any nearby objects and walk away from her until she calmed down. The rationale for this was that, previously, they would try to "talk her down" (i.e., providing soothing and reassuring statement such as, "That's OK," "Everybody loves you") sometimes for more than an hour. Unfortunately, there was no reduction in her tantrums with this procedure. The ignoring program was designed to avoid reinforcing her with attention for these tantrums. Despite these efforts, however, Carol's tantrums increased in frequency over time.

As a result of our assessments, it was determined that Carol's tantrums may have been occurring to escape or avoid academic demands. The previous calming-down procedure, as well as the ignoring program, may not have been effective because they both resulted in the temporary removal of tasks. Even though Carol's teachers and parents thought they were now not responding to her tantrums by ignoring them, they were in fact negatively reinforcing them. Carol's tantrums were reliably followed by the removal of academic materials and their associated demands, and this served to increase the frequency of her tantrums.

This example and the previous discussion illustrate how the term "ignoring" is often misused. Carol's case showed that when her parents and teachers thought they were ignoring her tantrums, they were actually responding in a very specific way. Our suggestion for *response-independent consequences* can be viewed as true ignoring (see Table 5-6). In other words, if one is to act as if the problem behavior is not occurring at all, then the consequence would involve no change in the environment or anyone else's behavior, with any changes being independent of the behavior problem itself. We have found that specifying ignoring in this way (i.e., pointing out that there are times when you might follow the behavior problem with a presumed reinforcer) makes it clear to those interacting with the student that we do not mean turning and walking away (unless, of course, you were about to do that anyway!).

Protect the Student

Several important issues must be addressed when recommending response-independent consequences for behavior problems. An important concern is protecting the student as well as those around him or her. Clearly, if the student is engaging in behavior that is dangerous, then some response is necessary. If, for example, a student begins to bang his or her head on a table hard enough to produce injury, someone will need to intervene. This intervention can involve such actions as placing something soft on the table to protect the student's head, moving the student away from the table, or holding his or her head up until he or she calms down. Similarly, if the student is engaging in behavior that could potentially hurt other students, then such actions as separating students or attempting to predict and prevent such situations is necessary.

Though such protective actions can be viewed as changing the way you behave as a consequence of the behavior, you can minimize the consequences of these crisis intervention procedures by limiting discussion

TABLE 5-6. Response-independent consequences

- Do protect the student
- Do not withdraw reinforcers for behavior problems
- Do not react to behavior problems

---

during these efforts, restricting efforts to "calm down" the student, and by returning to the activities started prior to the outburst. Any response on the part of the staff that is not absolutely essential for protecting the student (even if it seems to reduce the duration of these episodes) should be avoided.

Concerns about Using Response-Independent Consequences

An additional concern that has been expressed with this approach to reacting to behavior problems is the fear that occasionally people will respond in ways that are reinforcing to the student. Teachers, parents, and others worry that occasional positive consequences will serve to reinforce behavior problems intermittently, and will cause these behaviors to be maintained over time. In fact, using this procedure is likely to produce situations in which the behavior problem *is* followed by some positive consequence. Given that knowledge, should we be concerned?

Two factors mitigate the concern that behavior problems will increase or at least be maintained by this approach. The first issue is the *unpredictability* of the consequences. In order for a stimulus to reinforce any behavior, it should, optimally, reliably and predictably follow the response. Using our approach, no stimuli reliably or predictably follow the response. Sometimes a task might be removed because the teacher was doing that anyway, or sometimes the task will continue. Sometimes a parent will continue talking to their child, or at other times, they will be walking away. Because a particular consequence does not follow the behavior in any systematic fashion, the student should learn that this behavior has no effect on the environment.

A second related concept that also should allay the concerns of others involves the teaching of the functionally equivalent responses. Because you should be teaching the students another, more reliable way of getting what they want, they should not rely on their problem behavior for this purpose. Using response-independent consequences assumes that you are simultaneously teaching and reinforcing alternate responses as described previously.

Extinction Bursts

A positive aspect of this approach to intervention is being able to avoid "extinction bursts." When you remove reinforcement for a response, it is anticipated that the response that was previously reinforced will initially increase in frequency. This phenomenon is reliably observed in both animals (e.g., Millenson, 1967) and humans (e.g., Kelly, 1969). This is particularly problematic for the types of behaviors of interest here, because any increase in the frequency of behaviors such as aggression, self-injury, or tantrums could be quite dangerous. And, in fact, in animal studies, aggression is often observed in extinction conditions (e.g., Azrin, Hutchinson, & Hake, 1966; Hutchinson, Azrin, & Hunt, 1968).

However, *an extinction burst phenomenon has not been observed for most of our students.* One explanation may be that because we are providing the student with an alternate means of gaining the reinforcers that may actually be more efficient, they do not undergo the experience of having no response that is reinforced. Although the problem behavior is being reinforced less often, another response is provided to allow for more access to reinforcement. Again, this procedure is somewhat controversial, and those involved in intervention efforts should take extra care in translating this approach to their setting.

Summary

Figure 5-2 illustrates the intervention steps involved in functional communication training. Based on the assessments conducted prior to intervention, teachers, parents, and staff should teach a response that will serve the same function as the student's problem behavior. And, following the communication model adopted in this book, response-independent consequences should be used as a reaction to problem behavior. This combination of efforts has resulted in the successful intervention of a variety of behavior problems, in a variety of settings, and for a variety of individuals.

Conclusion

We have outlined in this chapter our efforts to teach students to use acceptable forms of communication to gain access to the things previously obtained with their problem behavior. Efforts were made in previous chapters to present necessary assessment and preintervention issues that directly impact on the potential success or failure of these interventions. As readers have surmised by now, even one aspect of an intervention program—teaching functionally equivalent responses—is a detailed and complex series of activities. And, the approach outlined here did not even attempt to describe in sufficient detail how to address adequately such issues as making meaningful changes in environments. Readers should refer to other excellent sources that specifically cover these approaches (e.g., see Meyer & Evans, 1989).

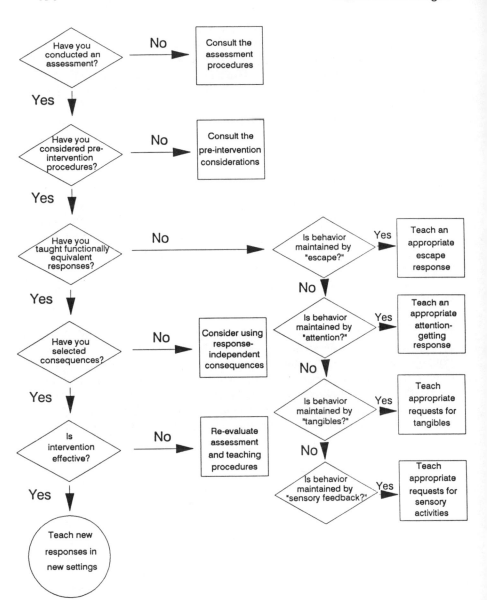

FIGURE 5-2. The complete intervention process.

Despite the varied issues we have presented here, it has always been surprising that *this approach to intervention has been successful in making meaningful changes in the lives of our students, even under less than optimal conditions.* Our experience has been that this is a robust intervention approach, one that has been effective even when all of the procedures are not followed exactly. We hope that this book provides readers with some assistance in dealing with difficult problems in difficult situations, and allows students to interact better with those around them.

The final chapter briefly outlines steps for designing an evaluation of your program. In addition, this section discusses some administrative issues important in providing optimal conditions for conducting interventions.

6

Administrative Issues and Evaluation Plans

In this final section, we briefly discuss several issues that will directly impact on the intervention process. Whether or not an intervention is successful depends in part on the support it receives from parents, teachers, clinicians, and administrators. Without considerable planning and effort on the part of these individuals, even the best-designed plans may not successfully result in meaningful behavior change. In addition, in order to estimate success and/or lack of progress, efforts at evaluation must be incorporated into each plan. Evaluation plans should be made from the beginning, and modified along the way when needed. Although we rarely design elaborate evaluation procedures, some measure of progress is necessary to assist in ongoing planning.

Addressing Administrative Issues

There are a number of administrative concerns that need to be addressed prior to designing any intervention. Although not presented here in detail, they are important enough to warrant some attention by those involved in designing interventions. Following are five administrative procedures that should be covered by agencies involved with interventions for severe behavior problems (Durand, Meyer, Janney, & Lanci, 1988).

1. *Develop a policy for the treatment of problem behavior.* Proper management strategy includes providing staff with a mission. This mission or goal could include a desire to intervene with challenging behavior, using only nonpainful or stigmatizing strategies. In addition, this strategy should

include specific guidelines for conducting such activities as assessment and intervention. General approaches to these activities should be in place before, for example, a crisis arises.

2. *Establish a Program Review Committee.* At a minimum, assessment and intervention decisions for severe behavior problems should be made by more than one or two persons. A group of persons with experience in areas such as skills training, medical assessment, and community training should be involved in all intervention planning. This should include *all* early efforts at even minimal changes in the student's program.

It appears that most guidelines are tied to the intrusiveness of the procedures used. In other words, approvals, special staff training, and consultations occur only after a decision has been made to intervene using highly restrictive interventions. It may be better to tie the level of approval to the seriousness of the behavior problem. *Any* intervention for behaviors such as self-injury or aggression should be approved by all parties involved (e.g., staff, parents, government agencies, etc.). The reason for this is that we should be concerned and involved in all programmatic efforts, not just those that involve restrictive or aversive components. If everyone is involved from the start (e.g., even with low-level differential reinforcement of other behavior [DRO] procedures or presumably minor environmental changes), then we may have more success with the less intrusive interventions.

3. *Ensure adequate staffing to implement suggested programs.* Although for some settings this is a faint goal, it is often the case that temporary measures can be made to provide extra assistance for interventions, even if it is on a part-time basis. It is best not to design a plan that cannot be adequately carried out by existing personnel.

4. *Coordinate monitoring efforts.* Especially for interventions occurring across different sites, monitoring the integrity of the intervention (i.e., are staff members carrying out the intervention as planned?) as well as the outcomes should be coordinated by one person. It is crucial that someone be responsible for seeing that the plans are progressing as expected, and that the student is receiving the best efforts possible.

5. *Provide mechanisms for continued staff development in proper assessment and intervention procedures.* Whether staff include teachers, parents, or others, continued effort should be made to ensure that all concerned have access to the latest knowledge concerning interventions for severe behavior problems. Because of the rapidly changing nature of this field, those who were trained in state-of-the-art assessment and intervention as little as 5 years ago, may not be aware of important advancements.

Again, this brief listing of important administrative concerns should serve to remind the reader that meaningful change cannot occur without administrative support (Durand & Kishi, 1987). And because this support is so important, it should be evaluated periodically, and should be explicitly planned to improve the chances for your program's success.

Designing an Evaluation Plan

Although many caregivers attempt to evaluate the effects of their interventions, often this process occurs in an ad hoc manner; after the intervention is already in place. It is important to plan the evaluation *prior to* the introduction of any changes in the environment or in the interactions with the student. Once an intervention is in place, it is often necessary to modify your evaluation strategy. However, planning before an intervention will improve the likelihood that the information gathered in this process will be useful.

The "basic ingredients" of an evaluation plan should include the following components (taken from Durand et al., 1988):

1. Projected completion dates, along with the duration that the program will be continued if there is no positive change in student behavior. It is also advised that an "emergency stop" criterion be determined, in cases where they may be an escalation of a behavior problem to dangerous levels.

2. Specific objectives for change in the targeted behavior(s), alternative behaviors, and changes in placement/living arrangements, expressed in terms that are observable and measurable.

3. The methods to be used and the schedule for the use of these methods.

4. The person responsible for the program.

5. The type of data and frequency of data collection necessary to be able to assess progress toward the desired objectives.

It is assumed that most readers are familiar with the basic aspects of designing a data collection and evaluation system. Therefore, we will not extensively discuss this issue here. For readers who would like more information about this topic, there are a number of books that would be helpful. One of the classic works in this area is by Beth Sulzer–Azaroff and G. Roy Mayer, *Applying Behavior-Analysis Procedures with Children and Youth* (1977). This book includes extensive discussion on topics such as "Selecting Observational Systems," and "Implementing Observational Systems." Other useful books that cover this topic in some detail include Meyer and Evans (1989), Rusch, Rose, and Greenwood (1988), Powers and Handleman (1984), Gaylord–Ross and Holvoet (1985), Gelfand and Hartmann (1984), and Kerr and Nelson (1989). Finally, readers may also wish general discussions, and useful articles on this topic include, Fabry and Cone (1980), Fowler (1986), Fuchs (1986), Scott and Goetz (1980), and White (1986).

Epilogue

Throughout this book there is an assumption that severe challenging behavior can be meaningfully reduced without resorting to painful or stigmatizing interventions. *All* interventions for the types of chronic problems discussed here require considerable effort. Modifications in programs, commitments by a variety of persons and agencies, and general training of service providers are just some of the practical aspects of successfully changing these behaviors. It is expected that with the types of efforts described in this book, and with the range of alternatives we currently have available, *all* students who exhibit challenging behaviors can be helped.

It has sometimes been said that there is no scientific evidence that all challenging behaviors can be reduced without occasionally using some painful interventions. One response to this argument is that *there are no data to suggest that any challenging behaviors require painful or stigmatizing interventions.* There are studies published that anecdotally describe that a variety of "nonaversive interventions" were tried and failed with a particular student, and that an intervention such as contingent electric shock reduced the frequency of his or her problem behaviors. However, studies do not exist demonstrating that a comprehensive intervention approach (such as described here) was attempted with proper consultation and that it failed to change the behaviors of the students participating.

With the increasing sophistication of our assessment procedures and the range of intervention options now available for challenging behavior (including functional communication training), there is reason to be enthusiastic about our ability to intervene. This positive, constructive view of persons with severe disabilities was articulated more generally 20 years ago by Bricker (1970):

> I wish to affirm my belief in the importance of the nervous system and to indicate a conviction that a host of events can do damage to it and to its functioning. However, only the failure of a perfectly valid, perfectly reliable, perfectly efficient program of training will convince me that the identification of the deficit is sufficient reason to stop trying to educate the child. (p. 20)

It is hoped that this book will provide one more reason to be optimistic about the humane treatment of persons with severe challenging behavior.

References

Alexander, F., & French, T. M. (1946). *Psychoanalytic therapy*. New York: Ronald.

Allen, L. D., & Iwata, B. A. (1980). Reinforcing exercise maintenance: Using existing high-rate activities. *Behavior Modification*, *4*, 337–354.

Alpert, C. L. (1984). *Milieu language intervention with mothers as teachers*. Unpublished doctoral dissertation, University of Kansas, Lawrence.

American Heritage Dictionary of the English Language. (1973). William Morris (Ed.) New college ed. Boston: Houghton Mifflin.

Anastasi, A. (1982). *Psychological testing*. (Fifth ed.) New York: Macmillan.

Atkinson, R. P., Jenson, W. R., Rovner, L., Cameron, S., Van Wagenen, L., & Petersen, B. P. (1984). Validation of the autism reinforcer checklist for children. *Journal of Autism and Developmental Disorders*, *14*, 429–433.

Ayllon, T. & Azrin, N. H. (1968). *The token economy*. New York: Appleton.

Azrin, N. H., Hutchinson, R. R., & Hake, D. J. (1966). Extinction-induced aggression. *Journal of the Experimental Analysis of Behavior*, *9*, 191–204.

Azrin, N. H., Kaplan, S. J., & Foxx, R. M. (1973). Autism reversal: Eliminating stereotypic self-stimulation of retarded individuals. *American Journal of Mental Deficiency*, *78*, 241–248.

Baer, D. M., & Wolf, M. M. (1970). The entry into natural communities of reinforcement. In R. Ulrich, T. Stachnik, & J. Mabry (Eds.), *Control of human behavior: From cure to prevention* (pp. 319–324). Glenview, IL: Scott, Foresman.

Baer, D. M., Wolf, M. M., & Risley, T. R. (1968). Some current dimensions of applied behavior analysis. *Journal of Applied Behavior Analysis*, *1*, 91–97.

Bailey, J. S., & Pyles, D. A. M. (1989). Behavioral diagnostics. In E. Cipani (Ed.), *The treatment of severe behavior disorders*. Washington: American Association on Mental Retardation.

Barlow, D. H., Hayes, S. C., & Nelson, R. O. (1984). *The scientist practitioner: Research and accountability in clinical and educational settings*. New York: Pergamon.

Barrett, C., Hampe, T. E., & Miller, L. (1978). Research on child psychotherapy. In S. Garfield & A. Bergin (Eds.), *Handbook of psychotherapy and behavior change* (pp. 411–436). New York: Wiley.

Bates, E., Camaioni, L., & Volterra, V. (1975). The acquisition of performatives prior to speech. *Merrill Palmer Quarterly*, *21*, 205–226.

Baumgart, D., Brown, L., Pumpian, I., Nisbet, J., Ford, A., Sweet, M., Messina, R., & Schroeder, J. (1982). Principle of partial participation and individualized adaptations in educational programs for severely handicapped students. *Journal of the Association for the Severely Handicapped, 7,* 17–27.

Baumgart, D., Vincent, L., Falvey, M., & Schroeder, J. (1982). Utilizing characteristics of a variety of current and subsequent least restrictive environments as factors in development of curricular content for severely handicapped students. In L. Brown, M. Falvey, D. Baumgart, I. Pumpian, J. Schroeder, & L. Gruenewald (Eds.), *Strategies for teaching chronological age-appropriate functional skills to adolescent and young adult severely handicapped students* (Vol. 9, Pt. 1). Madison: University of Wisconsin and Madison Metropolitan School District.

Bell, R. Q. (1968). A reinterpretation of the direction of effects in studies of socialization. *Psychological Review, 75,* 81–95.

Berkman, K. A., & Meyer, L. H. (1988). Alternative strategies and multiple outcomes in the remediation of severe self-injury: going "all out" nonaversively. *Journal of the Association for Persons with Severe Handicaps, 13,* 76–86.

Bijou, S. W., & Baer, D. M. (1961). *Child development I: A systematic and empirical theory.* New York: Appleton-Century-Crofts.

Bijou, S. W., Peterson, R. F., & Ault, M. H. (1968). A method to integrate descriptive and experimental field studies at the level of data and empirical concepts. *Journal of Applied Behavior Analysis, 1,* 175–191.

Bird, F., Dores, P. A., Moniz, D., & Robinson, J. (1989). Reducing severe aggressive and self-injurious behaviors with functional communication training: Direct, collateral and generalized results. *American Journal of Mental Retardation, 94,* 37–48.

Boakes, R. A. (1973). Response decrements produced by extinction and by response-independent reinforcement. *Journal of the Experimental Analysis of Behavior, 19,* 293–302.

Brackbill, Y., Adams, G., Crowell, D. H., & Gray, M. L. (1966). Arousal level in neonates and preschool children under continuous auditory stimulation. *Journal of Experimental Child Psychology, 4,* 178–188.

Bricker, W. A. (1970). Identifying and modifying behavioral deficits. *American Journal of Mental Deficiency, 75,* 16–21.

Brown, L., Long, E., Udvari–Solner, A., Davis, L., VanDeventer, P., Ahlgren, C., Johnson, F., Gruenewald, L., & Jorgensen, J. (1989a). The home school: Why students with severe intellectual disabilities must attend the schools of their brothers, sisters, friends, and neighbors. *Journal of the Association for Persons with Severe Handicaps, 14,* 1–7.

Brown, L., Long, E., Udvari–Solner, A., Schwarz, P., VanDeventer, P., Ahlgren, C., Johnson, F., Gruenewald, L., & Jorgensen, J. (1989b). Should students with severe intellectual disabilities be based in regular or special education classrooms in home schools? *Journal of the Association for Persons with Severe Handicaps, 14,* 8–12.

Brown, L., Nietupski, J., & Hamre–Nietupski, S. (1976). The criterion of ultimate functioning and public school services for severely handicapped students. In M. A. Thomas (Ed.), *Hey, don't forget about me: Education's investment in the severely, profoundly, and multiply handicapped* (pp. 2–15). Reston, VA: Council for Exceptional Children.

Bruner, J. S. (1973). Organization of early skilled action. *Child Development, 44,* 1–11.

Budd, K. S., & Kedesdy, J. H. (1989). Investigation of environmental factors in pediatric headache. *Headache, 29,* 1–5.

Carr, E. G. (1977). The motivation of self-injurious behavior: A review of some hypotheses. *Psychological Bulletin, 84,* 800–816.

Carr, E. G., & Durand, V. M. (1985a). Reducing behavior problems through functional communication training. *Journal of Applied Behavior Analysis, 18,* 111–126.

Carr, E. G., & Durand, V. M. (1985b). The social-communicative basis of severe behavior problems in children. In S. Reiss & R. R. Bootzin (Eds.), *Theoretical issues in behavior therapy* (pp. 219–254). New York: Academic.

Carr, E. G., & Lovaas, O. I. (1983). Contingent electric shock as a treatment for severe behavior problems. In S. Axelrod & J. Apsche (Eds.), *The effects of punishment on human behavior* (pp. 221–245). New York: Academic.

Carr, E. G., & McDowell, J. J., (1980). Social control of self-injurious behavior of organic etiology. *Behavior Therapy, 11,* 402–409.

Carr, E. G., Newsom, C. D., & Binkoff, J. A. (1976). Stimulus control of self-destructive behavior in a psychotic child. *Journal of Abnormal Child Psychology, 4,* 139–153.

Carr, E. G., Newsom, C. D., & Binkoff, J. A. (1980). Escape as a factor in the aggressive behavior of two retarded children. *Journal of Applied Behavior Analysis, 13,* 101–117.

Casey, R. J., & Berman, J. S. (1985). The outcome of psychotherapy with children. *Psychological Bulletin, 98,* 388–400.

Cataldo, M. F., & Harris, J. (1982). The biological basis for self-injury in the mentally retarded. *Analysis and Intervention in Developmental Disabilities, 2,* 21–39.

Catania, A. C. (1984). *Learning* (2nd ed.). Englewood Cliffs, NJ: Prentice-Hall.

Charlop, M. H., Kurtz, P. F., & Casey, F. G. (1989, May). *Using aberrant behaviors as reinforcers: The effects (and side-effects) of self-stimulation, delayed echolalia, and obsessive behavior.* Paper presented at the meeting of the Association for Behavior Analysis, Milwaukee.

Churchill, D. W. (1971). Effects of success and failure in psychotic children. *Archives of General Psychiatry, 25,* 208–214.

Cohen, H., Conroy, J. W., Frazer, D. W., Snelbecker, G. E., & Spreat, S. (1977). Behavioral effects of interinstitutional relocation of mentally retarded residents. *American Journal of Mental Deficiency, 82,* 12–18.

Cole, D. A., & Meyer, L. H. (1989). Impact of family needs and resources on the decision to seek out-of-home placement. *American Journal of Mental Retardation, 93,* 380–387.

Colman, R. S., Frankel, F., Ritvo, E., & Freeman, B. J. (1976). The effects of fluorescent and incandescent illumination upon repetitive behaviors in autistic children. *Journal of Autism and Childhood Schizophrenia, 6,* 157–162.

Conroy, J., Efthimiou, J., & Lemanowicz, J. (1982). A matched comparison of the developmental growth of institutionalized and deinstitutionalized mentally retarded clients. *American Journal of Mental Deficiency, 86,* 581–587.

Crimmins, D. B., & Durand, V. M. (in press). Assessment and evaluation. In I. M. Evans and B. Warren (Eds.), *Positive approaches to behavior change.* Albany, NY: Office of Mental Retardation and Developmental Disabilities.

Cronbach, L. J., Gleser, G., Nanda, H., & Rajaratnam, N. (1972). *The dependability of behavioral measurements: Theory of generalizability for scores and profiles.* New York: Wiley.

Datillo, J. (1986). Computerized assessment of preference for severely handicapped individuals. *Journal of Applied Behavior Analysis, 19,* 445–448.

Day, R. M., Johnson, W. L., & Schussler, N. G. (1986). Determining the communicative properties of self-injury: Research, assessment, & treatment implications. *Advances in learning and behavioral disabilities* (Vol. 5, pp. 117–139). Greenwich: CT: JAI.

Donnellan, A. M., & Mirenda, P. L. (1983). A model for analyzing instructional components to facilitate generalization for severely handicapped students. *Journal of Special Education, 17,* 317–331.

Donnellan, A. M., Mirenda, P. L., Mesaros, R. A., & Fassbender, L. L. (1984). Analyzing the communicative functions of aberrant behavior. *Journal of the Association for Persons with Severe Handicaps, 9,* 201–212.

Doss, L. S. (1988). *The effects of communication instruction on food stealing in adults with developmental disabilities.* Unpublished doctoral dissertation, University of Minnesota, Minneapolis.

Doss, S., & Reichle, J. (1989). Establishing communicative alternatives to the emission of socially motivated excess behavior: A review. *Journal of the Association for Persons with Severe Handicaps, 14*, 101–112.

Duker, P. (1975). Behaviour control of self-biting in a Lesch-Nyhan patient. *Journal of Mental Deficiency Research, 19*, 11–19.

Dunlap, G., & Johnson, J. (1985). Increasing the independent responding of autistic children with unpredictable supervision. *Journal of Applied Behavior Analysis, 18*, 227–236.

Dunlap, G., Koegel, R. L., Johnson, J., & O'Neill, R. E. (1987). Maintaining performance of autistic clients in community settings with delayed contingencies. *Journal of Applied Behavior Analysis, 20*, 185–191.

Dunlap, G., Plienis, A. J., & Williams, L. (1987). Acquisition and generalization of unsupervised responding: A descriptive analysis. *Journal of the Association for Persons with Severe Handicaps, 12*, 274–279.

Durand, V. M. (1982a). A behavioral/pharmacological intervention for the treatment of severe self-injurious behavior. *Journal of Autism and Developmental Disorders, 12*, 243–251.

Durand, V. M. (1982b). Analysis and intervention of self-injurious behavior. *Journal of the Association for the Severely Handicapped, 7*, 44–53.

Durand, V. M. (1983). Behavioral ecology of a staff incentive program: Effects on absenteeism and resident disruptive behavior. *Behavior Modification, 7*, 165–181.

Durand, V. M. (1984). *Attention-getting problem behavior: Analysis and intervention.* Unpublished doctoral dissertation, State University of New York, Stony Brook.

Durand, V. M. (1985). Employee absenteeism: A selective review of antecedents and consequences. *Journal of Organizational Behavior Management, 7*, 135–167.

Durand, V. M. (1986a). [Review of *Strategies for educating students with severe handicaps*]. *Journal of the Association for Persons with Severe Handicaps, 11*, 140–142.

Durand, V. M. (1986b). Self-injurious behavior as intentional communication. In K. D. Gadow (Ed.), *Advances in learning and behavioral disabilities* (Vol. 5, pp. 141–155). Greenwich, CT: JAI.

Durand, V. M. (1987) "Look Homeward Angel": A call to return to our (functional) roots. *Behavior Analyst, 10*, 299–302.

Durand, V. M. (1988). The Motivation Assessment Scale. In M. Hersen & A. Bellack (Eds.), *Dictionary of behavioral assessment techniques* (pp. 309–310). Elmsford, NY: Pergamon.

Durand, V. M., & Carr, E. G. (1982, November). *Contextual determinants of disruptive behavior.* Paper presented at the meeting of the Association for Advancement of Behavior Therapy, Chicago.

Durand, V. M., & Carr, E. G. (1985). Self-injurious behavior: Motivating conditions and guidelines for treatment. *School Psychology Review, 14*, 171–176.

Durand, V. M., & Carr, E. G. (1987). Social influences on "self-stimulatory" behavior: Analysis and treatment application. *Journal of Applied Behavior Analysis, 20*, 119–132.

Durand, V. M., & Carr, E. G. (1989). Operant learning methods with chronic schizophrenia and autism: Aberrant behavior. In J. L. Matson (Ed.), *Chronic schizophrenia and adult autism: Issues on diagnosis, assessment, and psychological treatment* (pp. 231–273). New York: Springer.

Durand, V. M., & Carr, E. G. (in press). Functional communication training to reduce challenging behavior: Maintenance and application in new settings. *Journal of Applied Behavior Analysis.*

Durand, V. M., & Crimmins, D. B. (1983, October). *The Motivation Assessment Scale: A preliminary report on an instrument which assesses the functional significance of children's deviant behavior.* Paper presented at the meeting of the Berkshire Association for Behavior Analysis and Therapy, Amherst, MA.

Durand, V. M., & Crimmins, D. B. (1987) Assessment and treatment of psychotic speech in an autistic child. *Journal of Autism and Developmental Disorders, 17*, 17–28.

Durand, V. M., & Crimmins, D. B. (1988). Identifying the variables maintaining self-injurious behavior. *Journal of Autism and Developmental Disorders, 18*, 99–117.

Durand, V. M., Crimmins, D. B., Caulfield, M., & Taylor, J. (1989). Reinforcer assessment I: Using problem behavior to select reinforcers. *Journal of the Association for Persons with Severe Handicaps, 14*, 113–126.

Durand, V. M., & Kishi, G. (1987). Reducing severe behavior problems among persons with dual sensory impairments: An evaluation of a technical assistance model. *Journal of the Association for Persons with Severe Handicaps, 12*, 2–10.

Durand, V. M., Meyer, L. H., Janney, R., & Lanci, A. (1988). *New York State Education Department behavior management guidelines.* Albany: New York State Education Department.

Dyer, K. (1987). The competition of autistic stereotyped behavior with usual and specially assessed reinforcers. *Research in Developmental Disabilities, 8*, 607–626.

Eason, L. J., White, M. J., & Newsom, C. (1982). Generalized reduction of self-stimulatory behavior: An effect of teaching appropriate play to autistic children. *Analysis and Intervention in Developmental Disabilities, 2*, 157–169.

Edelson, S. M., Taubman, M. T., & Lovaas, O. I. (1983). Some social contexts of self-destructive behavior. *Journal of Abnormal Child Psychology, 11*, 299–312.

Evans, I. M., & Meyer, L. H. (1985). *An educative approach to behavior problems.* Baltimore: Paul H. Brookes.

Eyman, R. K., & Borthwick, S. A. (1980). Patterns of care for mentally retarded persons. *Mental Retardation, 18*, 63–66.

Eyman, R. K., & Call, T. (1977). Maladaptive behavior and community placement of mentally retarded persons. *American Journal of Mental Deficiency, 82*, 137–144.

Fabry, B. D., & Cone, J. D. (1980). Auto-graphing: A one step approach to collecting and graphing data. *Education and Treatment of Children, 3*, 361–368.

Favell, J. E. (1973). Reduction of stereotypies by reinforcement of toy play. *Mental Retardation, 11*, 21–23.

Favell, J. E., Azrin, N. H., Baumeister, A. A., Carr, E. G., Dorsey, M. F., Forehand, R., Foxx, R. M., Lovaas, O. I., Rincover, A., Risley, T. R., Romanczyk, R. G., Russo, D. C., Schroeder, S. R., & Solnick, J. V. (1982). The treatment of self-injurious behavior. *Behavior Therapy, 13*, 529–554.

Favell, J. E., McGimsey, J. F., & Schell, R. M. (1982). Treatment of self-injury by providing alternate sensory activities. *Analysis and Intervention in Developmental Disabilities, 2*, 83–104.

Ferster, C. B. (1965). Classification of behavioral pathology. In L. Krasner & L. P. Ullmann (Eds.), *Research in behavior modification*, (pp. 6–26). New York: Holt, Rinehart, & Winston.

Ferster, C. B., Culbertson, S., & Boren, M. C. (1975). *Behavior principles* (3rd ed.). Englewood Cliffs, NJ: Prentice-Hall.

Forness, S. R., Guthrie, D., & MacMillan, D. L. (1982). Classroom environments as they relate to mentally retarded children's observable behavior. *American Journal of Mental Deficiency, 87*, 259–265.

Fowler, S. A. (1986). Peer-monitoring and self-monitoring: Alternatives to traditional teacher management. *Exceptional Children, 52*, 573–581.

Foxx, R. M., & Bechtel, D. R. (1983). Overcorrection: A review and analysis. In S. Axelrod & J. Apsche (Eds.), *The effects of punishment on human behavior*, (pp. 133–220). New York: Academic.

Foxx, R. M., McMorrow, M. J., Bittle, R. G., & Bechtel, D. R. (1986). The successful treatment of a dually-diagnosed deaf man's aggression with a program that included contingent electric shock. *Behavior Therapy, 17*, 170–186.

Foxx, R. M., Plaska, T. G., & Bittle, R. G. (1986). Guidelines for the use of contingent electric shock to treat aberrant behavior. In M. Hersen, A. Bellack, & P. Miller (Eds.), *Progress in behavior modification* (Vol. 20, pp. 1–33). New York: Academic.

Friedman, P. R. (1975). Legal regulation of applied behavior analysis in mental institutions and prisons. *Arizona Law Review, 17*, 39–64.

Fuchs, L. S. (1986). Monitoring progress among mildly handicapped pupils: Review of current practice and research. *Remedial and Special Education, 7*, 5–12.

Gardner, W. I., Cole, C. L., Davidson, D. P., & Karan, O. C. (1986). Reducing aggression in individuals with developmental disabilities: An expanded stimulus control, assessment, and intervention model. *Education and Training of the Mentally Retarded, 21*, 3–12.

Gardner, W. I., Karan, O. C., & Cole, C. L. (1984). Assessment of setting events influencing functional capacities of mentally retarded adults with behavior difficulties. In A. S. Halpern & M. J. Fuhrer (Eds.), *Functional assessment in rehabilitation* (pp. 171–185). Baltimore: Brookes.

Gaylord–Ross, R. (1980). A decision model for the treatment of aberrant behavior in applied settings. In W. Sailor, B. Wilcox, & L. Brown (Eds.), *Methods of instruction for severely handicapped students* (pp. 135–158). Baltimore: Brookes.

Gaylord–Ross, R. J., Haring, T. G., Breen, C., & Pitts–Conway, V. (1984). The training and generalization of social intervention skills with autistic youth. *Journal of Applied Behavior Analysis, 17*, 229–247.

Gaylord–Ross, R. J. & Holvoet, J. F. (1985). *Strategies for educating students with severe handicaps.* Boston: Little, Brown

Gedye, A. (1989). Extreme self-injury attributed to frontal lobe seizures. *American Journal on Mental Retardation, 94*, 20–26.

Gelfand, D. M., & Hartmann, D. P. (1984). *Child behavior analysis and therapy* (2nd ed.). New York: Pergamon.

Gibson, C. A., Walker, H. M., Crimmins, D. B., & Griggs, P. A. (1988). Resource manual. In C. F. Calkins & H. M. Walker (Eds.), *Enhancing employment outcomes habilitation training program: Improving the social competence of workers with developmental disabilities in integrated employment settings.* Kansas City, MO: UMKC Institute for Human Development.

Gillberg, C., & Steffenburg, S. (1987). Outcome and prognostic factors in infantile autism and similar conditions: A population-based study of 46 cases followed through puberty. *Journal of Autism and Developmental Disorders, 17*, 273–287.

Goetz, L., Schuler, A., & Sailor, W. (1983). Motivational considerations in teaching language to severely handicapped students. In M. Hersen, V. B. Van Hasselt, & J. L. Matson (Eds.), *Behavior therapy for the developmentally and physically disabled* (pp. 57–77). New York: Academic.

Goldiamond, I. (1983, May). Discussion. In I. Goldiamond (Chair), *The interdependence of formal, basic, and applied behavior analysis: Can the bell toll for just one?* Symposium conducted at the meeting of the Association for Behavior Analysis, Milwaukee.

Goldstein, A. P., & Glick, B. (1987). *Aggression replacement training: A comprehensive intervention for aggressive youth.* Champaign, IL: Research.

Green, C. W., Reid, D. H., White, L. K., Halford, R. C., Brittain, D. P., & Gardner, S. M. (1988). Identifying reinforcers for persons with profound handicaps: Staff opinion versus systematic assessment of preference. *Journal of Applied Behavior Analysis, 21*, 31–43.

Groden, G. (1989). A guide for conducting a comprehensive behavioral analysis of a target behavior. *Journal of Behavior Therapy and Experimental Psychiatry, 20*, 37–49.

Guess, D. (1980). Methods in communication instruction for severely handicapped persons. In W. Sailor, B. Wilcox, & L. Brown (Eds.), *Methods of instruction for severely handicapped students* (pp. 195–225). Baltimore: Paul H. Brookes.

Guess, D., Helmstetter, E., Turnbull, H. R., III, & Knowlton, S. (1987). *Use of aversive procedures with persons who are disabled: A historical review and critical analysis, TASH Monograph Series, No. 2.* Seattle: Association for Persons with Severe Handicaps.

Guess, D., & Siegel–Causey, E. (1985). Behavioral control and education of severely handicapped students: Who's doing what to whom? And why? In D. Bricker & J. Filler (Eds.), *Severe mental retardation: From theory to practice* (pp. 230–244). Reston, VA: Council for Exceptional Children.

Halderman v. Pennhurst State School and Hospital, 446 F. Supp. 1295 (E. D. Pa. 1977), *aff'd. in part, rev'd. in part,* 612 F. 2d 84 (3rd Cir. 1979), *rev'd. and remanded,* 451 U. S. 1 (1981).

Haley, J. (1963). *Strategies of psychotherapy.* New York: Grune & Stratton.

Hall, T., Laitinen, R., & Mozzoni, M. (1985, May). *The reduction of aggression through student-directed choice of demand/no demand settings.* Paper presented at the annual meeting of the Association for Behavior Analysis, Columbus, OH.

Halle, J. (1988). Adopting the natural environment as the context of training. In S. N. Calculator & J. L. Bedroscan (Eds.), *Communication assessment for adults with mental retardation* (pp. 155–185). San Diego: College Hill.

Halle, J. W., Baer, D. H., & Spradlin, J. E. (1981). An analysis of teacher's generalized use of delay in helping children: A stimulus control procedure to increase language use in handicapped children. *Journal of Applied Behavior Analysis, 14,* 389–409.

Hanley–Maxwell, C., Rusch, F. R., Chadsey–Rusch, J., & Renzaglia, A. (1986). Reported factors contributing to job termination of individuals with severe disabilities. *Journal of the Association for Persons with Severe Handicaps, 11,* 45–52.

Haring, T. G., Neetz, J. A., Lovinger, L., Peck, C. A., & Semmel, M. I. (1987). Effects of four modified incidental teaching procedures to create opportunities for communication. *Journal of the Association for Persons with Severe Handicaps, 12,* 218–226.

Harris, S. L. (1975). Teaching language to nonverbal children with emphasis on problems of generalization. *Psychological Bulletin, 82,* 565–580.

Harris, S. L., & Ersner–Hershfield, R. (1978). Behavioral suppression of seriously disruptive behavior in psychotic and retarded patients: A review of punishment and its alternatives. *Psychological Bulletin, 85,* 1352–1375.

Hart, B. (1981). Pragmatics: How language is used. *Analysis and Intervention in Developmental Disabilities, 1,* 299–313.

Hart, B. (1985). Environmental techniques that may facilitate generalization and acquisition. In S. F. Warren & A. K. Rogers–Warren (Eds.), *Teaching functional language* (pp. 63–88). Baltimore: University Park.

Hartmann, D. P., Roper, B. L., & Gelfand, D. M. (1977). An evaluation of alternative modes of child psychotherapy. In B. Lahey & A. E. Kazdin (Eds.), *Advances in clinical child psychology* (Vol. 1, pp. 1–46). New York: Plenum.

Hawkins, R. P. (1986). Selection of target behaviors. In R. O. Nelson & S. C. Hayes (Eds.), *Conceptual foundations of behavioral assessment* (pp. 331–385). New York: Guilford.

Hayes, R. P. (1987). Training for work. In D. C. Cohen & A. M. Donnellan (Eds.), *Handbook of autism and pervasive developmental disorders* (pp. 360–370). New York: Wiley.

Hayes, S. C., Nelson, R. O., & Jarrett, R. B. (1987). The treatment utility of assessment: A functional approach to evaluating assessment quality. *American Psychologist, 42,* 963–974.

Haynes, S. N., & Horn, W. F. (1982). Reactivity in behavioral observations: A methodological and conceptual critique. *Behavioral Assessment, 4,* 369–385.

Herbert, E. W., Pinkston, E. M., Hayden, M. L., Sajwaj, T. E., Pinkston, S., Cordua, G., & Jackson, C. (1973). Adverse effects of differential parental attention. *Journal of Applied Behavior Analysis, 6,* 15–30.

Holz, W. C., Azrin, N. H., & Allyon, T. (1963). Elimination of behavior of mental patients by response-produced extinction. *Journal of the Experimental Analysis of Behavior, 6,* 407–412.

Homme, L. E. C., de Baca, P., Devine, J. V., Steinhorst, R., & Rickert, E. J. (1963). Use of the Premack principle in controlling the behavior of nursery school children. *Journal of the Experimental Analysis of Behavior, 6,* 544.

Horner, R. H., & Billingsley, F. (1988). The effect of competing behavior on the generalization and maintenance of adaptive behavior in applied settings. In R. H. Horner, G. Dunlap, & R. L. Koegel (Eds.), *Generalization and maintenance: Life-style changes in applied settings* (pp. 197–220). Baltimore: Brookes.

Horner, R. H., & Budd, C. M. (1985). Acquisition of manual sign use: Collateral reduction of maladaptive behavior, and factors limiting generalization. *Education and Training of the Mentally Retarded, 20,* 39–47.

Hung, D. W. (1978). Using self-stimulation as reinforcement for autistic children. *Journal of Autism and Childhood Schizophrenia, 8,* 355–366.

Hunt, P., Alwell, M., & Goetz, L. (1988). Acquisition of conversational skills and the reduction of inappropriate social interaction behaviors. *Journal of the Association for Persons with Severe Handicaps, 13,* 20–27.

Hutchinson, R. R., Azrin, N. H., & Hunt, G. M. (1968). Attack produced by intermittent reinforcement of a concurrent operant response. *Journal of the Experimental Analysis of Behavior, 11,* 489–495.

Hutt, C., & Vaizey, M. J. (1966). Differential effects of group density on social behavior. *Nature, 209,* 1371–1372.

Iwata, B. A., Dorsey, M. F., Slifer, K. J., Bauman, K. E., & Richman, G. S. (1982). Toward a functional analysis of self injury. *Analysis and Intervention in Developmental Disabilities, 2,* 3–20.

Jacobson, J. W. (1982). Problem behavior and psychiatric impairment within a developmentally disabled population I: Behavior frequency. *Applied Research in Mental Retardation, 3,* 121–139.

James, W. (1893). *Psychology.* New York: Holt.

Kearney, C. A., & Silverman, W. K. (1988, November). *Measuring the function of school refusal behavior: The school refusal assessment scale.* Paper presented at the meeting of the Association for the Advancement of Behavior Therapy, New York.

Kelly, J. F. (1969). *Extinction induced aggression in humans.* Unpublished master's thesis, Southern Illinois University, Carbondale, IL.

Kent, L. (1974). *Language acquisition program for severely retarded.* Champaign, IL: Research.

Kerr, M. M., & Nelson, C. M. (1989). *Strategies for managing behavior problems in the classroom* (2nd ed.). Columbus, OH: Charles E. Merrill

Koegel, R. L., & Covert, A. (1972). The relationship of self-stimulation to learning in autistic children. *Journal of Applied Behavior Analysis, 5,* 381–387.

Koegel, R. L., Dyer, K., & Bell, L. K. (1987). The influence of child-preferred activities on autistic children's social behavior. *Journal of Applied Behavior Analysis, 20,* 243–252.

Koegel, R. L., Egel, A. L., & Williams, J. A. (1980). Behavioral contrast and generalization across settings in the treatment of autistic children. *Journal of Experimental Child Psychology, 30,* 422–437.

Koegel, R. L., & Johnson, J. (1989). Motivating language use in autistic children. In G. Dawson (Ed.), *Autism* (pp. 310–325). New York: Guilford.

Koegel, R. L., & Mentis, M. (1985). Motivation in child autism: Can they or won't they? *Journal of Child Psychology and Psychiatry, 26,* 185–191.

Koegel, R. L., & Williams, J. A. (1980). Direct versus indirect response-reinforcer relationships in teaching autistic children. *Journal of Abnormal Child Psychology, 8,* 537–547.

Konarski, E. A., Crowell, C. R., Johnson, M. R., & Whitman, T. L. (1982). Response deprivation, reinforcement, and instrumental academic performance in an EMR classroom. *Behavior Therapy, 13*, 94–102.

Konarski, E. A., Johnson, M. R., Crowell, C. R., & Whitman, T. L. (1981). An alternative approach to reinforcement for applied researchers: Response deprivation. *Behavior Therapy, 12*, 653–666.

Layng, T. V. J., & Andronis, P. T. (1984). Toward a functional analysis of delusional speech and hallucinatory behavior. *Behavior Analyst, 7*, 139–156.

LaVigna, G. W., & Donnellan, A. M. (1986). *Alternatives to punishment: Nonaversive strategies for solving behavior problems*. New York: Irvington.

Leigland, S. (1984). On "setting events" and related concepts. *Behavior Analyst, 7*, 41–45.

Lennox, D. B., Miltenberger, R. G., Spengler, P., & Erfanian, N. (1988). Decelerative treatment practices with persons who have mental retardation: A review of five years of the literature. *American Journal on Mental Retardation, 92*, 492–501.

Litt, M. D., & Schreibman, L. (1982). Stimulus-specific reinforcement in the acquisition of receptive labels by autistic children. *Analysis and Intervention in Developmental Disabilities, 1*, 171–186.

Lovaas, O. I., Freitag, G., Gold, V. J., & Kassorla, I. C. (1965). Experimental studies in childhood schizophrenia: Analysis of self-destructive behavior. *Journal of Experimental Child Psychology, 2*, 67–84.

Lovaas, O. I., Koegel, R., Simmons, J. Q., & Long, J. S. (1973). Some generalization and follow-up measures on autistic children in behavior therapy. *Journal of Applied Behavior Analysis, 6*, 131–166.

Lovaas, O. I., & Simmons, J. Q. (1969). Manipulation of self-destruction in three retarded children. *Journal of Applied Behavior Analysis, 2*, 143–157.

Luiselli, J. K., & Townsend, N. M. (1980). Effects of intermittent punishment in behavior modification programs with children: A review. *Journal of Corrective and Social Psychiatry, 26*, 200–205.

MacDonald, J. D. (1985). Language through conversation: A model for intervention with language delayed persons. In S. F. Warren & A. K. Rogers–Warren (Eds.), *Teaching functional language* (pp. 91–122). Baltimore: University Park.

Martin, P. L., & Foxx, R. M. (1973). Victim control of the aggression of an institutionalized retardate. *Journal of Behavior Therapy and Experimental Psychiatry, 4*, 161–165.

Mason, S. A., McGee, G. G., Farmer-Dougan, V., & Risley, T. R. (1989). A practical strategy for ongoing reinforcer assessment. *Journal of Applied Behavior Analysis, 22*, 171–179.

Matson, J. L., & Kazdin, A. E. (1981). Punishment in behavior modification: Pragmatic, ethical, and legal issues. *Clinical Psychology Review, 1*, 197–210.

Meyer, L. H., & Evans, I. M. (1986). Modification of excess behavior: An adaptive and functional approach for educational and community contexts. In R. H. Horner, L. H. Meyer, & H. D. Fredericks (Eds.), *Education of learners with severe handicaps: Exemplary service strategies* (pp. 315–350). Baltimore: Brookes.

Meyer, L. H., & Evans, I. M. (1989). *Nonaversive intervention for behavior problems: A manual for home and community*. Baltimore: Brookes.

Meyer, L. H., & Putnam, J. (1988). Social integration. In V. B. Van Hasselt, P. S. Strain, & M. Hersen (Eds.), *Handbook of developmental and physical disabilities* (pp. 107–133). New York: Pergamon.

Michael, J. L. (1982). Distinguishing between discriminative and motivational functions of stimuli. *Journal of the Experimental Analysis of Behavior, 37*, 149–155.

Millenson, J. R. (1967). *Principles of behavior analysis*. New York: Macmillan.

Minuchin, S. (1974). *Families and family therapy*. Cambridge, MA: Harvard University.

Mitchell, W. S., & Stoffelmayr, B. E. (1973). Application of the Premack principle to the behavioral control of extremely inactive schizophrenics. *Journal of Applied Behavior Analysis, 6,* 419–423.

Mullins, M., & Rincover, A. (1985). Comparing autistic and normal children along dimensions of reinforcement maximization, stimulus sampling, and responsiveness to extinction. *Journal of Experimental Child Psychology, 40,* 350–374.

Mulligan, M., Lacy, L., & Guess, D. (1982). Effects of massed, distributed, and spaced trial sequencing on severely handicapped students' performance. *Journal of the Association for the Severely Handicapped, 7,* 48–61.

Murphy, G. H., & Wilson, B. (1981). Long-term outcome of contingent shock treatment for self-injurious behavior. In P. Mittler (Ed.), *Frontiers of knowledge in mental retardation.* (pp. 303–311). London: IASSMD.

Neel, R. S., & Billingsley, F. F. (1989). *Impact: A functional curriculum handbook for students with moderate to severe disabilities.* Baltimore: Brookes.

Neel, R. S., Billingsley, F. F., McCarty, F., Symonds, D., Lambert, C., Lewis-Smith, N., & Hanashira, R. (1983). *Innovative model program for autistic children and their teachers.* Unpublished manuscript, University of Washington, Seattle.

Nelson, R. O., & Hayes, S. C. (Eds.). (1986). *Conceptual foundations of behavioral assessment.* New York: Guilford.

O'Neill, R. E., Horner, R. H., Albin, R. W., Storey, K., & Sprague, J. R. (1989). *Functional analysis: A practical assessment guide.* University of Oregon: Research and Training Center on Community-Referenced Nonaversive Behavior Management.

Osborne, J. G. (1969). Free-time as a reinforcer in the maintenance of classroom behavior. *Journal of Applied Behavior Analysis, 2,* 113–118.

Pace, G., Ivancic, M., Edwards, G., Iwata, B., & Page, T. (1985). Assessment of stimulus preferences and reinforcer values with profoundly retarded individuals. *Journal of Applied Behavior Analysis, 18,* 249–255.

Patterson, G. R. (1982). *Coercive family process.* Eugene, OR: Castalia.

Paul, G. L. (1967). Insight versus desensitization in psychotherapy two years after termination. *Journal of Consulting Psychology, 31,* 333–348.

Peck, C. A. (1985). Increasing opportunities for social control by children with autism and severe handicaps: Effects on student behavior and perceived classroom climate. *Journal of the Association for Persons with Severe Handicaps, 10,* 183–193.

Pirsig, R. M. (1974). *Zen and the art of motorcycle maintenance.* New York: William Morrow.

Plato (348 B. C. /1960). *The Laws* (A. E. Taylor, Trans.), London: J. M. Dent.

Podboy, J. W., & Mallery, W. A. (1977). Caffeine reduction and behavior change in the severely retarded. *Mental Retardation, 15,* 40.

Powers, M. D., & Handleman, J. S. (1984). *Behavioral assessment of severe developmental disabilities.* Rockville, MD: Aspen.

Premack, D. (1959). Toward empirical behavior laws I. : Positive reinforcement. *Psychological Review, 66,* 219–233.

Premack, D. (1965). Reinforcement theory. In D. Levine (Ed.), *Nebraska symposium on motivation.* Lincoln: University of Nebraska.

Premack, D. (1971). Catching up with common sense or two sides of a generalization: Reinforcement and punishment. In R. Glase (Ed.), *The nature of reinforcement.* New York: Academic.

Prokasy, W. F. (1965). Classical eyelid conditioning: Experimenter operations, task demands, and response shaping. In W. F. Prokasy (Ed.), *Classical conditioning: A symposium* (pp. 208–225). New York: Appleton-Century-Crofts.

Rachlin, H. (1970). *Introduction to modern behaviorism.* San Francisco: W. H. Freeman.

Reichle, J., & Karlan, G. (1985). The selection of an augmentative system in communication intervention: A critique of decision rules. *Journal of the Association for Persons with Severe Handicaps, 10*, 146–156.

Reichle, J. E., & Yoder, D. E. (1979). Assessment and early stimulation of communication in the severely and profoundly mentally retarded. In R. L. York & E. E. Edgar (Eds.), *Teaching the severely handicapped (Vol. 4*, pp. 180–218). Seattle: American Association for the Severely/Profoundly Handicapped.

Reid, D. II., & Hurlbut, B. (1977). Teaching nonvocal communication skills to multihandicapped retarded adults. *Journal of Applied Behavior Analysis, 10*, 591–603.

Renzaglia, A., & Bates, P. (1983). Teaching socially appropriate behavior: In search of social competence. In M. E. Snell (Ed.), *Systematic instruction of the moderately and severely handicapped* (2nd ed., pp. 314–356). Columbus, OH: Charles E. Merrill.

Repp, A. C., Barton, L. E., & Gottlieb, J. (1983). Naturalistic studies of institutionalized profoundly or severely mentally retarded persons: The relationship of density and behavior. *American Journal of Mental Deficiency, 87*, 441–447.

Repp, A. C., Felce, D., & Barton, L. E. (1988). Basing the treatment of stereotypic and self-injurious behaviors on hypotheses of their causes. *Journal of Applied Behavior Analysis, 21*, 281–289.

Rescorla, R. A. (1967). Pavlovian conditioning and its proper control procedures. *Psychological Review, 74*, 71–80.

Rescorla, R. A., & Skucy, J. C. (1969). Effect of response-independent reinforcers during extinction. *Journal of Comparative and Physiological Psychology, 67*, 381–389.

Reynolds, G. S. (1961). Behavioral contrast. *Journal of the Experimental Analysis of Behavior, 4*, 57–71.

Rheingold, H. L. (1969). The social and socializing infant. In D. A. Goslin (Eds.), *Handbook of socialization theory and research* (pp. 779–790). Chicago: Rand McNally.

Rincover, A. (1978). Sensory extinction: A procedure for eliminating self-stimulatory behavior in psychotic children. *Journal of Abnormal Child Psychology, 6*, 299–310.

Rincover, A., Cook, R., Peoples, A., & Packard, D. (1979). Sensory extinction and sensory reinforcement principles for programming multiple adaptive behavior change. *Journal of Applied Behavior Analysis, 12*, 221–233.

Rincover, A., & Devany, J. (1982). The application of sensory extinction procedures to self-injury. *Analysis and Intervention in Developmental Disabilities, 2*, 67–81.

Rojahn, J., Mulick, J. A., McCoy, D., & Schroeder, S. R. (1978). Setting effects, adaptive clothing, and the modification of head banging and self-restraint in two profoundly retarded adults. *Behavior Analysis and Modification, 2*, 185–196.

Romanczyk, R. G. (in press). Aversive conditioning as a component of comprehensive treatment: The impact of etiological factors on clinical decision making. In S. Harris & J. Handleman (Eds.), *Life threatening behavior: Aversive vs. non-aversive interventions.* New Brunswick, NJ: Rutgers University.

Romanczyk, R. G., Colletti, G., & Plotkin, R. (1980). Punishment of self-injurious behavior: Issues of behavior analysis, generalization, and the right to treatment. *Child Behavior Therapy, 2*, 37–54.

Romanczyk, R. G., Kistner, J. A., & Plienis, A. (1982). Self-stimulatory and self-injurious behavior: Etiology and treatment. In J. J. Steffen & P. Karoly (Eds.), *Advances in child behavioral analysis and severe psychopathology* (pp. 189–254). Lexington MA: Lexington Books.

Rousseau, J. J. (1762/1979). *Emile* (A. Bloom, Trans.) New York: Basic Books.

Rusch, F. R., Rose, T., & Greenwood, C. R. (1988). *Introduction to behavior analysis in special education.* Englewood Cliffs, NJ: Prentice-Hall.

Sailor, W., Guess, D., Goetz, L., Schuler, A., Utley, B., & Baldwin, M. (1980). Language and severely handicapped persons: Deciding what to teach to whom. In W. Sailor, B.

Wilcox, & L. Brown (Eds.), *Methods of instruction for severely handicapped students* (pp. 71–105). Baltimore: Brookes.

Saunders, R., & Sailor, W. (1979). A comparison of three strategies of reinforcement on two-choice learning problems with severely retarded children. *American Association for Education of the Severely and Profoundly Handicapped Review, 4,* 323–333.

Schalock, R. L., Harper, R. S., & Genung, T. (1981). Community integration of mentally retarded adults: Community placement and program success. *American Journal of Mental Deficiency, 85,* 478–488.

Scheerenberger, R. C. (1981). Deinstitutionalization: Trends and difficulties. In R. H. Bruininks, C. E. Meyers, B. B. Sigford, & K. C. Lakin (Eds.), *Deinstitutionalization and community adjustment of mentally retarded people* (Monograph No. 4, pp. 3–13). Washington: American Association on Mental Deficiency.

Schiefelbusch, R. L. (1978). *Language intervention strategies.* Baltimore: University Park.

Schiefelbusch, R. L. (1980). A discussion of special issues. In R. L. Schielbusch (Eds.), *Nonspeech language and communication: Analysis and Intervention.* Baltimore: University Park.

Schopler, E., Brehm, S., Kinsbourne, M., & Reichler, R. J. (1971). Effect of treatment structure on development in autistic children. *Archives of General Psychiatry, 24,* 415–421.

Schreibman, L., & Carr, E. G. (1978). Elimination of echolalic responding to questions through the training of a generalized verbal response. *Journal of Applied Behavior Analysis, 11,* 453–463.

Schroeder, S. R., & Henes, C. (1978). Assessment of progress of institutionalized and deinstitutionalized retarded adults: A matched control comparison. *Mental Retardation, 16,* 147–148.

Schuler, A. L., & Goetz, L. (1981). The assessment of severe language disabilities: Communicative and cognitive considerations. *Analysis and Intervention in Developmental Disabilities, 1,* 333–346.

Schuler, A. L., Peck, C. A., Tomlinson, C., & Theimer, R. K. (1984). Assessment. In C. A. Peck, A. L. Schuler, C. Tomlinson, R. K. Theimer, T. Haring, & M. I. Semmel (Eds.), *The social competence curriculum project: A guide to instructional programming for social and communicative interactions* (pp. 22–106). Santa Barbara, CA: University of California—Santa Barbara Special Education Research Institute.

Schwartz, I. S., Anderson, S. R., & Halle, J. W. (1989). Training teachers to use naturalistic time delay: Effects on teacher behavior and on language use of students. *Journal of the Association for Persons with Severe Handicaps, 14,* 48–57.

Scott, L. C., & Goetz, E. M. (1980). Issues in the collection of in-class data by teachers. *Education and Treatment of Children, 3,* 65–71.

Shapiro, M. (1974). Legislating the control of behavior control: Autonomy and the coercive use of organic therapies. *Southern California Law Review, 47,* 237–338.

Shatz, M., & Gelman, R. (1973). The development of communication skills: Modifications in the speech of young children as a function of listener. *Monographs of the Society for Research in Child Development, 38,* 1–38.

Shodell, M. J., & Reiter, H. H. (1968). Self-mutilative behavior in verbal and nonverbal schizophrenic children. *Archives of General Psychiatry, 19,* 453–455.

Sidman, M. (1989). *Coercion and its fallout.* Boston: Authors Cooperative.

Singer, G. H. S., Close, D. W., Irvin, L. K., Gersten, R., & Sailor, W. (1984). An alternative to the institution for young people with severely handicapping conditions in a rural community. *Journal of the Association for the Severely Handicapped, 9,* 251–261.

Smith, M. D. (1985). Managing the aggressive and self-injurious behavior of adults disabled by autism. *Journal of the Association for Persons with Severe Handicaps, 10,* 228–232.

Smith, M. D., & Coleman, D. (1986). Managing the behavior of adults with autism in the job setting. *Journal of Autism and Developmental Disorders, 16,* 145–154.

Snow, C. (1972). Mother's speech to children learning language. *Child Development, 43*, 549–565.

Sparrow, S. S., Balla, D. A., & Cicchetti, D. V. (1984). *Vineland Adaptive Behavior Scales*, Circle Pines, MN: American Guidance Service.

Stokes, T. F., & Baer, D. M. (1977). An emplicit technology of generalization. *Journal of Applied Behavior Analysis, 10*, 349–367.

Sulzer–Azaroff, B., & Mayer, G. R. (1977). *Applying behavior-analysis procedures with children and youth*. New York: Holt, Rinehart, & Winston.

Sulzer–Azaroff, B., & Mayer, G. R. (1986). *Achieving educational excellence: Using behavioral strategies*. New York: Holt, Rinehart, & Winston.

Sulzer–Azaroff, B., & Reese, E. P. (1982). *Applying behavior analysis: A program for developing professional competence*. New York: Holt, Rinehart & Winston.

Swahn, O. (1988). Effect of parent-administered interruption on excessive climbing in a 2-year-old developmentally disabled girl. *Scandinavian Journal of Behaviour Therapy, 17*, 17–24.

Talkington, L. W., Hall, S., & Altman, R. (1971). Communication deficits and aggression in the mentally retarded. *American Journal of Mental Deficiency, 76*, 235–237.

Tharp, R. G., & Wetzel, R. J. (1969). *Behavior modification in the natural environment*. New York: Academic.

The Association for Persons with Severe Handicaps. (1981, November). Resolution on intrusive interventions. *TASH Newsletter, 7*, 1–2.

Touchette, P. E. (1968). The effects of graduated stimulus change on the acquisition of a simple discrimination in severely retarded boys. *Journal of the Experimental Analysis of Behavior, 11*, 39–48.

Touchette, P. E., MacDonald, R. F., & Langer, S. N. (1985). A scatter plot for identifying stimulus control of problem behavior. *Journal of Applied Behavior Analysis, 18*, 343–351.

Turnbull, H. R. (Ed.) (1981). *The least restrictive alternative: Principle and practice*. Washington: American Association on Mental Deficiency.

Van Houten, R., Axelrod, S., Bailey, J. S., Favell, J. E. Foxx, R. M., Iwata, B. A., & Lovaas, O. I. (1988). The right to effective behavioral treatment. *Behavior Analyst, 11*, 111–114.

Varela, J. S. (1977). Social technology. *American Psychologist, 32*, 914–923.

Voeltz, L. M., Evans, I. M., Derer, K. R., & Hanashiro, R. (1983). Targeting excess behavior for change: A clinical decision model for selecting priority goals in educational contexts. *Child and Family Behavior Therapy, 5*, 17–35.

Voeltz, L. M., Evans, I. M., Freedland, K., & Donellon, S. (1982). Teacher decision making in the selection of educational priorities for severely handicapped children. *Journal of Special Education, 16*, 179–198.

Wachtel, P. L. (1977). *Psychoanalysis and behavior therapy: Toward an integration*. New York: Basic Books.

Wacker, D. P., Berg, W. K., Wiggins, B., Muldoon, M., & Cavanaugh, J. (1985). Evaluation of reinforcer preferences for profoundly handicapped students. *Journal of Applied Behavior Analysis, 18*, 173–178.

Wahler, R. G. (1975). Some structural aspects of deviant child behavior. *Journal of Applied Behavior Analysis, 8*, 27–42.

Wahler, R. G., & Fox, J. J. (1981). Setting events in applied behavior analysis: Toward a conceptual and methodological expansion. *Journal of Applied Behavior Analysis, 14*, 327–338.

Weeks, M., & Gaylord–Ross, R. (1981). Task difficulty and aberrant behavior in severely handicapped students. *Journal of Applied Behavior Analysis, 14*, 449–463.

White, O. R. (1986). Precision teaching—precision learning. *Exceptional Children, 52*, 522–534.

Wieseler, N. A., Hanson, R. H., Chamberlain, T. P., & Thompson, T. (1985). Functional taxonomy of stereotypic and self-injurious behavior. *Mental Retardation, 23,* 230–234.

Williams, J. A., Koegel, R. L., & Egel, A. L. (1981). Response-reinforcer relationships and improved learning in autistic children. *Journal of Applied Behavior Analysis, 14,* 53–60.

Wolery, M. (1978). Self-stimulatory behavior as a basis for devising reinforcers. *AAESPH Review, 3,* 23–29.

Wolery, M., Kirk, K., & Gast, D.L. (1985). Stereotypic behavior as a reinforcer: Effects and side effects. *Journal of Autism and Developmental Disorders, 15,* 149–161.

Wolff, P. H. (1969). The natural history of crying and other vocalizations in early infancy. In B. M. Foss (Eds.). *Determinants of infant behavior* (Vol. 4, pp. 81–109). London: Methuen.

Wuerch, B. B., & Voeltz, L. M. (1982). *Longitudinal leisure skills for severely handicapped learners: The Ho'onanea curriculum component.* Baltimore: Brookes.

Yoder, D. E., & Calculator, S. (1981). Some perspectives on intervention strategies for persons with developmental disorders. *Journal of Autism and Developmental Disorders, 11,* 107–123.

Zigler, E., & Balla, D. (1977). Personality factors in the performance of the retarded: Implications for clinical assessment. *Journal of the American Academy of Child Psychiatry, 16,* 19–37.

Zlotnik, D. (1981). First do no harm: Least restrictive alternative analysis and the right of mental patients to refuse treatment. *West Virginia Law Review, 83,* 376–448.

Appendices: Blank Forms

COMMUNICATIVE RESPONSE "FORM" CHECKLIST

Student's Name:_____ Date:_____

Expected Response to Others: _____
(e.g., assistance, tangibles) _____

Communicative Response: _____
(include form, e.g., verbal) _____

Circle YES or NO for each of the questions below.

1. Is this response one that can be easily   YES   NO
   taught to the student (i.e., within a few
   days or weeks)?

2. Is this response one that could be   YES   NO
   understood by someone not familiar
   with the student?

3. Is this response appropriate for those   YES   NO
   situations in which most problem
   behaviors seem to occur?

4. Is this response one that will be   YES   NO
   responded to appropriately by other
   people?

5. If used appropriately, would other   YES   NO
   people *not* find this response annoying?

If you answered NO to any of the above questions, then a
different communicative response (I.e., form and/or modality)
should be considered.

MOTIVATION ASSESSMENT SCALE

Name _____ Rater _____ Date _____

Behavior Description _____

Setting Description _____

Instructions: The **Motivation Assessment Scale** is a questionnaire designed to identify those situations in which an individual is likely to behave in certain ways. From this information, more informed decisions can be made concerning the selection of appropriate reinforcers and treatments. To complete the **Motivation Assessment Scale**, select one behavior that is of particular interest. It is important that you identify the behavior *very specifically*. *Aggressive*, for example, is not as good a description as *hits his sister*. Once you have specified the behavior to be rated, read each question carefully and circle the *one* number that best describes your observations of this behavior.

QUESTIONS

ANSWERS

	Never	Almost Never	Seldom	Half the Time	Usually	Almost Always	Always
1. Would the behavior occur continuously, over and over, if this person was left alone for long periods of time? (For example, several hours.)	0	1	2	3	4	5	6
2. Does the behavior occur following a request to perform a difficult task?	0	1	2	3	4	5	6
3. Does the behavior seem to occur in response to your talking to other persons in the room?	0	1	2	3	4	5	6
4. Does the behavior ever occur to get a toy, food, or activity that this person has been told that he or she can't have?	0	1	2	3	4	5	6

	Never	Almost Never	Seldom	Half the Time	Usually	Almost Always	Always
	0	1	2	3	4	5	6

5. Would the behavior occur repeatedly, in the same way, for very long periods of time, if no one was around? (For example, rocking back and forth for over an hour.)

Never 0	Almost Never 1	Seldom 2	Half the Time 3	Usually 4	Almost Always 5	Always 6

6. Does the behavior occur when any request is made of this person?

Never 0	Almost Never 1	Seldom 2	Half the Time 3	Usually 4	Almost Always 5	Always 6

7. Does the behavior occur whenever you stop attending to this person?

Never 0	Almost Never 1	Seldom 2	Half the Time 3	Usually 4	Almost Always 5	Always 6

8. Does the behavior occur when you take away a favorite toy, food, or activity?

Never 0	Almost Never 1	Seldom 2	Half the Time 3	Usually 4	Almost Always 5	Always 6

9. Does it appear to you that this person enjoys performing the behavior? (It feels, tastes, looks, smells, and/or sounds pleasing.)

Never 0	Almost Never 1	Seldom 2	Half the Time 3	Usually 4	Almost Always 5	Always 6

10. Does this person seem to do the behavior to upset or annoy you when you are trying to get him or her to do what you ask?

Never 0	Almost Never 1	Seldom 2	Half the Time 3	Usually 4	Almost Always 5	Always 6

11. Does this person seem to do the behavior to upset or annoy you when you are not paying attention to him or her? (For example, if you are sitting in a separate room, interacting with another person.)

Never 0	Almost Never 1	Seldom 2	Half the Time 3	Usually 4	Almost Always 5	Always 6

12. Does the behavior stop occurring shortly after you give this person the toy, food or activity he or she has requested?

Never 0	Almost Never 1	Seldom 2	Half the Time 3	Usually 4	Almost Always 5	Always 6

13. When the behavior is occurring, does this person seem calm and unaware of anything else going on around him or her?

Never 0	Almost Never 1	Seldom 2	Half the Time 3	Usually 4	Almost Always 5	Always 6

14. **Does the behavior stop occurring shortly after (one to five minutes) you stop working or making demands of this person?**

Never	Almost Never	Seldom	Half the Time	Usually	Almost Always	Always
0	1	2	3	4	5	6

15. **Does this person seem to do the behavior to get you to spend some time with him or her?**

Never	Almost Never	Seldom	Half the Time	Usually	Almost Always	Always
0	1	2	3	4	5	6

16. **Does the behavior seem to occur when this person has been told that he or she can't do something he or she had wanted to do?**

Never	Almost Never	Seldom	Half the Time	Usually	Almost Always	Always
0	1	2	3	4	5	6

Sensory	Escape	Attention	Tangible
1. _____	2. _____	3. _____	4. _____
5. _____	6. _____	7. _____	8. _____
9. _____	10. _____	11. _____	12. _____
13. _____	14. _____	15. _____	16. _____

Total score = _____ _____ _____ _____

Mean score = _____ _____ _____ _____

Relative ranking = _____ _____ _____ _____

1986 V. Mark Durand, Ph.D.

COMMUNICATIVE RESPONSE MODALITY CHECKLIST

Student's Name:_____ **Date:**_____

Respondent's Name:_____

1. Does the student use one of the following methods of communication on a regular basis? (if more than one is used, circle the preferred method)

   VERBAL   SIGN/GESTURAL   SYMBOLIC   NO

   If one of the above methods is circled, this may be the modality used for the communicative response. If NO is circled, go to question #2.

2. Does the student use one or more verbal responses to communicate on an occasional basis (e.g., "cookie," "no")?

   YES   NO

   If YES, then the communicative response might be verbal. If NO, go on to question #3.

3. Does the student use one or more signs or understandable gestures to communicate on an occasional basis?

   YES   NO

   If YES, then the communicative response might be signed/gestural. If NO, go on to question #4.

4. Does the student use one or more verbal symbolic forms of communication to communicate on an occasional basis (e.g., points to pictures in a picture book)?

   YES   NO

   If YES, then the communicative response may be symbolic. If NO, go on to question #5.

5. Is one method of communication being emphasized in speech/language training?

   YES   NO

   If YES, then the communicative response may be in the modality currently used in training. If previous speech/language training has been unsuccessful with all modalities, attempt simple gestures or symbols to start.

FUNCTIONAL COMMUNICATION TRAINING
DATA SHEET

Student's Name: _____   **Date:** _____

Training days [date]	Number of training trials attempted	Number of successful trials	Best response	Frequency of problem behavior

Index